Biologics for the Treatment of Allergic Diseases

Editor

LANNY J. ROSENWASSER

IMMUNOLOGY AND ALLERGY CLINICS OF NORTH AMERICA

www.immunology.theclinics.com

November 2020 • Volume 40 • Number 4

ELSEVIER

1600 John F. Kennedy Boulevard • Suite 1800 • Philadelphia, Pennsylvania, 19103-2899

http://www.theclinics.com

IMMUNOLOGY AND ALLERGY CLINICS OF NORTH AMERICA Volume 40, Number 4

November 2020 ISSN 0889-8561, ISBN-13: 978-0-323-77730-8

Editor: Katerina Heidhausen
Developmental Editor: Kristen Helm

Immunology and Allergy Clinics of North America (ISSN 0889–8561) is published quarterly by Elsevier Inc., 360 Park Avenue South, New York, NY 10010-1710. Months of issue are February, May, August, and November. Periodicals postage paid at New York, NY and additional mailing offices. Subscription prices are $344.00 per year for US individuals, $623.00 per year for US institutions, $100.00 per year for US students and residents, $423.00 per year for Canadian individuals, $100.00 per year for Canadian students, $791.00 per year for Canadian institutions, $447.00 per year for international individuals, $791.00 per year for international institutions, $220.00 per year for international students. To receive student/resident rate, orders must be accompanied by name of affiliated institution, date of term, and the *signature* of program/residency coordinator on institution letterhead. Orders will be billed at individual rate until proof of status is received. Foreign air speed delivery is included in all *Clinics* subscription prices. All prices are subject to change without notice. **POSTMASTER**: Send address changes to *Immunology and Allergy Clinics of North America,* Elsevier Health Sciences Division, Subscription Customer Service, 3251 Riverport Lane, Maryland Heights, MO 63043. **Customer Service: 1-800-654-2452 (U.S. and Canada); 314-447-8871 (outside U.S. and Canada). Fax: 314-447-8029. E-mail: journalscustomerservice-usa@elsevier.com (for print support); journalsonlinesupport-usa@elsevier.com (for online support).**

Reprints. For copies of 100 or more, of articles in this publication, please contact the Commercial Reprints Department, Elsevier Inc., 360 Park Avenue South, New York, New York 10010-1710. Tel. 212-633-3874, Fax: 212-633-3820, E-mail: reprints@elsevier.com.

Immunology and Allergy Clinics of North America is covered in MEDLINE/PubMed (Index Medicus), Current Contents/Life Sciences, Science Citation Index, ISI/BIOMED, Chemical Abstracts, and EMBASE/Excerpta Medica.

Contributors

EDITOR

LANNY J. ROSENWASSER, MD
Professor Allergy/Immunology, Department of Medicine, UMKC School of Medicine, Kansas City, Missouri, USA

AUTHORS

IGNACIO J. ANSOTEGUI, MD, PhD
Department of Allergy and Immunology, Hospital Quironsalud Bizkaia, Erandio-Bilbao, Spain

DIEGO BAGNASCO, MD
Allergy and Respiratory Diseases, IRCCS Policlinico San Martino, University of Genoa, Genova, Genoa, Italy

MARK BOGUNIEWICZ, MD
Professor, Division of Allergy-Immunology, Department of Pediatrics, National Jewish Health and University of Colorado School of Medicine, Denver, Colorado, USA

LARRY BORISH, MD
Professor of Medicine and Microbiology, Departments of Medicine and Microbiology, Asthma and Allergic Disease Center, University of Virginia Health Systems, Charlottesville, Virginia, USA

KANWALJIT K. BRAR, MD
Allergy and Immunology, Department of Pediatrics, NYU Grossman School of Medicine, New York, New York, USA

MARCO CAMINATI, MD
Department of Medicine, Allergy and Clinical Immunology Section, University Hospital GB Rossi, University of Verona and Verona University Hospital, Verona, Italy

LINDA COX, MD
Associate Professor of Medicine, Department of Medicine Nova Southeastern University, Casper, Wyoming, USA

SANDRA GONZÁLEZ DÍAZ, MD
Centro Regional de Excelencia CONACYT/WAO en Alergia Asma e Inmunologia Clìnica, Hospital Universitario, Facultad de Medicina, Universidad Autonoma de Nuevo Leon, Monterrey, Nuevo Leon, Mèxico; San Francisco Centro de Especialistas Médicos

WILLIAM ESCHENBACHER, MD
Department of Medicine, Asthma and Allergic Disease Center, University of Virginia Health Systems, Charlottesville, Virginia, USA

ALEX D. FEDERMAN, MD
Professor of Medicine, Division of General Internal Medicine, Icahn School of Medicine at Mt. Sinai, New York, New York, USA

FERNANDO HOLGUIN, MD
Professor of Medicine, Division of Pulmonary Sciences and Critical Care Medicine, University of Colorado School of Medicine, Aurora, Colorado, USA

SANDHYA KHURANA, MD
Professor of Medicine, Division of Pulmonary and Critical Care Medicine, University of Rochester School of Medicine and Dentistry, Rochester, New York, USA

ALICE KNOEDDLER, MD
Department of Medicine, Asthma and Allergic Disease Center, University of Virginia Health Systems, Charlottesville, Virginia, USA

BRUCE J. LANSER, MD
Allergy and Immunology, Department of Pediatrics, National Jewish Health, Denver, Colorado, USA

RUNG-CHI LI, DO
Department of Medicine, Asthma and Allergic Disease Center, University of Virginia Health Systems, Charlottesville, Virginia, USA

CLAUDIO LUNARDI, MD
Chair of Allergy and Clinical Immunology, Department of Medicine, University Hospital GB Rossi, University of Verona, Verona, Italy

JONATHAN J. LYONS, MD
Translational Allergic Immunopathology Unit, Laboratory of Allergic Diseases, National Institutes of Health, Bethesda, Maryland, USA

ERIC MACY, MD, MS, FAAAAI
Southern California Permanente Medical Group, Kaiser Permanente Southern California, San Diego Medical Center, San Diego, California, USA

BRYAN MARTIN, DO
Department of Medicine, The Ohio State University, Columbus, Ohio, USA

DEAN D. METCALFE, MD
Mast Cell Biology Section, Laboratory of Allergic Diseases, National Institute of Allergy and Infectious Diseases, National Institutes of Health, Bethesda, Maryland, USA

ANNA NOWAK-WEGRZYN, MD, PhD
Allergy and Immunology, Department of Pediatrics, NYU Grossman School of Medicine, New York, New York, USA; Department of Pediatrics, Gastroenterology and Nutrition, Collegium Medicum, University of Warmia and Mazury, Olsztyn, Poland

BIANCA OLIVIERI, MD
Department of Medicine, University Hospital GB Rossi, University of Verona, Verona, Italy

JOSE ANTONIO ORTEGA-MARTELL, MD
Universidad Autónoma del Estado de Hidalgo, Pachuca, Hidalgo, México

MARIA ISABEL ROJO, MD
Allergy Service, Juarez Hospital, Mexico City, Mexico

LANNY J. ROSENWASSER, MD
Professor Allergy/Immunology, Department of Medicine, UMKC School of Medicine, Kansas City, Missouri, USA

MARIO SÁNCHEZ-BORGES, MD
Allergy and Clinical Immunology Department, Centro Médico Docente La Trinidad, Allergy and Clinical Immunology Department, Clínica El Avila, Caracas, Venezuela

AMANDA SCHNEIDER, MD
Allergy and Immunology, Department of Pediatrics, NYU Long Island School of Medicine, Mineola, New York, USA

GIANENRICO SENNA, MD
Department of Medicine, Allergy and Clinical Immunology School, University of Verona, Asthma Center and Allergy Unit, Verona University Hospital, Verona, Italy

SUNITA SHARMA, MD
Associate Professor of Medicine, Division of Pulmonary Sciences and Critical Care Medicine, University of Colorado School of Medicine, Aurora, Colorado, USA

MATTHEW STRAESSER, MD
Department of Medicine, Asthma and Allergic Disease Center, University of Virginia Health Systems, Charlottesville, Virginia, USA

LUCIANA KASE TANNO, MD, PhD
Hospital Sírio-Libanês, University Hospital of Montpellier, WHO Collaborating Centre on Scientific Classification Support, Montpellier, France; Sorbonne Université, INSERM UMR-S 1136, IPLESP, Equipe EPAR, Paris, France

ELISA TINAZZI, MD
Department of Medicine, University Hospital GB Rossi, University of Verona, Verona, Italy

ANDREA VIANELLO, MD
Respiratory Pathophysiology Division, University of Padua, Padua, Italy; Dipartimento di Scienze CardioToracoVascolari e Sanit Pubblica, Padova, Padua, Italy

JUAN WISNIVESKY, MD
Professor of Medicine, Division of General Internal Medicine, Icahn School of Medicine at Mt. Sinai, New York, New York, USA

Contents

Allergic rhinitis (AR), most presentations of nasal polyposis (NP), and many presentations of chronic rhinosinusitis are type 2^{high} disorders characterized by expression of interleukin (IL)-4, IL-5, and IL-13. Neutralization of IgE with anti-IgE (omalizumab) has proven efficacy in AR. Similarly, in addition to anti-IgE, blockade of IL-5/IL-5 (mepolizumab, reslizumab, benralizumab) and dual blockade of IL-4 and IL-13 with anti-IL-4R (dupilumab) have demonstrated efficacy in NP. However, these agents are expensive and future studies are essential to evaluate cost effectiveness in comparison with current medical and surgical therapies. This article reviews biologics as potential interventions in AR, chronic rhinosinusitis, and NP.

By selectively targeting specific steps of the immune inflammation cascade, biologic drugs for severe asthma have substantially contributed to increase the standard of care, to reduce drug-related morbidity. and most importantly to ameliorate patients' quality of life. Upcoming molecules are going to provide a chance for severe phenotypes besides Th2 high through the interaction with epithelial and innate immunity. Some practical aspects including optimal treatment duration, the possibility of a dose treatment modulation, the place and relevance of ICS in best responders are still under debate. Long-term safety, especially when interacting with innate immunity needs to be further investigated.

Asthma-chronic obstructive pulmonary disease (COPD) overlap (ACO) defines a subgroup of patients with asthma who have persistent airflow obstruction or patients with COPD who may exhibit variable airflow limitation and/or evidence of type 2 inflammation. Additional investigations are needed to determine whether ACO represents a distinct disorder with unique underlying pathophysiology, whether ACO patients should be managed differently from those with asthma or COPD, and whether the diagnosis affects long-term outcomes. This article presents the data about the clinical features of ACO, the current information regarding the underlying pathophysiology of the syndrome, and current understanding of therapeutic options.

Food allergy is increasingly prevalent and poses a life-threatening risk to those afflicted. The health care costs associated with food allergies are also increasing. Current and emerging treatments for food allergies aim at protecting against reactions caused by accidental ingestion and increasing the food allergen reaction threshold, although this protection is often temporary. In the future, ideal biologic therapies would target key mediators of the type II immune pathway, essential in development of the atopic march to prevent development of food allergies. Biologics offering long-term protection against allergic reactions to food are needed, and several agents are already in development.

Atopic dermatitis (AD) is a common chronic inflammatory skin disease that has become a global health problem. The pathophysiology of AD includes both skin barrier and immune abnormalities, with type 2 immune deviation central to several clinical phenotypes and underlying endotypes. Recognition of the persistent nature and systemic aspects of AD provides a rationale for treatment with a biologic. Dupilumab has been approved for patients 6 years of age and older with moderate to severe AD. Monoclonal antibodies are in phase 3 trials and may become part of a precision medicine approach to AD.

This article reviews biologic treatments that are currently applied for the treatment of severe chronic urticaria. Monoclonal anti–immunoglobulin E (omalizumab) is effective and safe in many patients, but accessibility and cost constitute barriers to its wider use. Questions on the optimal duration of the treatment and possible symptom recurrences after discontinuing the drug are still raised. A discussion is presented about several other biologics currently under investigation with potential to be incorporated in the near future in patients with severe chronic urticaria.

Several biologic therapies and new devices are emerging as potential preventive treatment of anaphylaxis. However, adrenaline (epinephrine) is still the first-line treatment of any type of anaphylaxis. Biologic drugs, such as omalizumab, although not US Food and Drug Administration approved for anaphylaxis, have been used as therapeutic adjuvants in the preventive treatment of anaphylaxis, but cost-effectiveness should be considered individually.

Biologic and other therapies used for the treatment of immune-mediated hypersensitivity conditions, and in people with immune-mediated hypersensitivity, can trigger a wide variety of immune-related adverse drug reactions and immunologically mediated drug hypersensitivities. These range from acute-onset immunoglobulin E–mediated allergies to delayed-onset T-cell–mediated hypersensitivities. Certain therapeutic and diagnostic agents can directly activate mast cells. Biologic agents used to treat immune-mediated hypersensitivity can also globally upregulate or downregulate the immune system leading to pathologic reactions, including cytokine storm and hypogammaglobulinemia.

Eosinophil-associated diseases are characterized by a common pathogenetic background, represented by eosinophil-led inflammation and overexpression of interleukin (IL)-5. IL-5 and its receptor are excellent therapeutic targets for eosinophil-associated diseases. Three monoclonal antibodies targeting IL-5 currently are available: mepolizumab and reslizumab block circulating IL-5 preventing the binding to its receptor, whereas benralizumab binds to IL-5 receptor α. They have a steroid-sparing effect in eosinophil disorders, such as eosinophilic granulomatosis with polyangiitis, hypereosinophilic syndrome, allergic bronchopulmonary aspergillosis, eosinophilic esophagitis, and chronic eosinophilic pneumonia. The biotechnological drugs targeting IL-5 are promising therapies; however, further studies are needed.

Mast cells are tissue-resident allergic effector cells that cause many symptoms associated with IgE–mediated immediate hypersensitivity reactions. Beginning with allergen-specific therapy over a century ago, biologics have been used to target mast cells in patients in order to reduce allergic symptoms and reactions. This review discusses the history and current outlook of the use of biologics in mast cell–associated diseases and reactions.

Allergic diseases represent some of the most chronic and costly chronic conditions. Medical management may require long-term pharmacotherapy, which is often associated with poor adherence. Although medications provide symptomatic control, they do not modify the allergic disease.

Patients may prefer disease-modifying treatments that provide lasting benefits after discontinuation. To date, allergy immunotherapy is the only proved disease modification therapy associated with lasting benefits after discontinuation. However, allergy immunotherapy safety and efficacy has only been established in allergic rhinitis, mild to moderate asthma, and some patients with atopic dermatitis.

IMMUNOLOGY AND ALLERGY CLINICS OF NORTH AMERICA

FORTHCOMING ISSUES

February 2021
Climate Change and Allergy
Jae-Won Oh, *Editor*

May 2021
Food Allergy
Amal Assa'ad, *Editor*

August 2021
Skin Allergy
Susan T. Nedorost, *Editor*

RECENT ISSUES

August 2020
Immunodeficiencies
Mark Ballow and Elena Perez, *Editors*

May 2020
Rhinosinusitis
Sandra Y. Lin, *Editor*

February 2020
Update on Immunotherapy for Aeroallergens, Foods, and Venoms
Linda S. Cox and Anna Nowak-Wegrzyn, *Editors*

SERIES OF RELATED INTEREST

Medical Clinics
http://medical.theclinics.com/

THE CLINICS ARE AVAILABLE ONLINE!
Access your subscription at:
www.theclinics.com

Preface

A New Era in the Treatment of Allergic Disorders

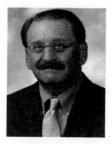

Lanny J. Rosenwasser, MD
Editor

Biologics have revolutionized medical therapy in the past 2 decades. Allergic Diseases have benefited from this revolution as a variety of biologics have impacted all categories of allergic diseases. Anticytokines directed at type 2 immunity has helped in the treatment of all allergic conditions covered in this issue ranging from Allergic Rhinitis to Asthma to Atopic Dermatitis to Food Allergy and others. Obviously, the ravages of COVID-19 on processes involved in biologic treatment are a consideration, but current thinking suggests such therapies should not be affected by the pandemic.[1]

Lanny J. Rosenwasser, MD
Department of Medicine
UMKC School of Medicine
Kansas City, MO 64106, USA

E-mail address:
lrosenwasser334@gmail.com

REFERENCE

1. Morais-Almeida M, Aguiar R, Martin B, et al. COVID-19, asthma, and biological therapies: what we need to know. World Allergy Organ J 2020;13:100126.

Biologics for the Treatment of Allergic Rhinitis, Chronic Rhinosinusitis, and Nasal Polyposis

William Eschenbacher, MD[a], Matthew Straesser, MD[a],
Alice Knoeddler, MD[a], Rung-chi Li, DO[a], Larry Borish, MD[a,b],*

KEYWORDS

- Allergic rhinitis • Chronic rhinosinusitis • Nasal polyposis • Type 2 inflammation
- Eosinophils • Interleukins • IgE

KEY POINTS

- Allergic rhinitis, most presentations of nasal polyposis (NP), and many presentations of chronic rhinosinusitis (CRS) are type 2^{high} (interleukin [IL]-4^{high}, IL-5^{high}, IL-13^{high}) inflammatory diseases of the upper airway.
- Allergic rhinitis is mediated in large part by IgE and responds to IgE-targeting biologics.
- Efficacy of biologics in CRS without nasal polyposis is theoretically plausible but no efficacy studies have been performed.
- Biologics that target IgE, IL-5, and the IL-4 receptor (the receptor for IL-4 and IL-13) have all demonstrated efficacy in the treatment of NP.
- Studies are essential to evaluate the cost effectiveness of biologics in these disorders and their proper placement in therapy in comparison with available medical and surgical therapies.

INTRODUCTION

Allergic rhinitis (AR), many presentations of chronic rhinosinusitis (CRS), and most presentations of CRS with nasal polyposis (NP) are recognized as type 2 (T2) inflammatory diseases. These $T2^{high}$ inflammatory conditions are characterized by infiltration with eosinophils, basophils, mast cells, and other inflammatory cells and are recognized by the robust expression of cytokines associated with T-helper 2 (Th2) effector

[a] Department of Medicine, Asthma and Allergic Disease Center, University of Virginia Health Systems, Charlottesville, VA 22908-1355, USA; [b] Department of Microbiology, Asthma and Allergic Disease Center, University of Virginia Health Systems, Charlottesville, VA 22908-1355, USA
* Correspondence: MR4 Building Room 5041a, 409 Lane Road, Charlottesville, VA 22908.
E-mail address: lb4m@virginia.edu

Immunol Allergy Clin N Am 40 (2020) 539–547
https://doi.org/10.1016/j.iac.2020.06.001
0889-8561/20/© 2020 Elsevier Inc. All rights reserved.

immunology.theclinics.com

cells, specifically interleukin (IL)-4, IL-5, and IL-13. The term T2^{high} is now the preferred term for this inflammatory phenotype, in recognition of the numerous additional sources of Th2 effector cytokines, such as innate lymphoid 2 cells (ILC2s), eosinophils, mast cells, and numerous others. Although not specifically developed for T2 diseases of the upper airway, recognition of the roles of these T2 cytokines in driving the presence and severity of these conditions has led to the exploration of biologics that were developed for other T2 conditions (atopic dermatitis and asthma) as therapeutic options. This article reviews the use of biologics as potential interventions in AR, CRS, and NP.

BIOLOGICS IN THE TREATMENT OF ALLERGIC RHINITIS

AR is in large part an allergic disorder mediated by specific IgE directed against aeroallergens. However, AR is also a quintessential T2 disorder with this T2 cytokine expression being driven not only by allergen-specific Th2 effector lymphocytes but also by nasal stromal cells and recruited immune cells. It is this T2^{high} state driving the recruitment of basophils, mast cells, eosinophils, ILC2 cells, and numerous other inflammatory cells that along with the allergic/IgE-mediated component is responsible for the full expression of the upper airway, ocular, and lower airway symptoms. To the extent that AR is driven by aeroallergen-specific IgE, it is the cross-linking of surface IgE and the consequent mast and basophil degranulation that leads to the release of the vasoactive and other proinflammatory mediators that strongly contribute to the symptoms of AR. Omalizumab (humanized anti-IgE antibody) binds to IgE and thereby captures IgE antibodies and prevents their binding to the high-affinity receptor (FcεRI). Reduced binding of IgE leads to the disassociation of the high-affinity receptor and thereby dramatically decreases the expression of FcεRI on mast cells and basophils, and on antigen-presenting cells. This decreased availability of surface IgE on antigen-presenting dendritic cells and B cells interferes with IgE antibody-mediated facilitated antigen capture and thereby contributes to the amelioration of Th2 activation and the T2^{high} state.[1] All of these effects make omalizumab an inviting treatment of AR refractory to the conventional therapies of oral antihistamines, intranasal steroids, and intranasal antihistamines/cromolyn.

Although only Food and Drug Administration (FDA)-approved for the treatment of moderate-to-severe persistent asthma and chronic idiopathic urticaria, omalizumab has been extensively studied in the treatment of AR as a direct and as an add-on therapy. In a recent review and meta-analysis by Yu and colleagues,[2] 83 articles were identified regarding omalizumab for the treatment of AR and, of these, 16 were randomized controlled trials. These latter 16 studies were used as the focus of their analysis and these involved a total of 3458 patients (1931 experimental and 1527 control subjects). Their analysis showed statistically significant differences between the omalizumab and control groups in daily nasal symptom score, daily ocular symptom score, daily nasal medication symptom scores, proportion of days of emergency drug use, rhinoconjunctivitis-specific quality of life questionnaires, and overall evaluation (**Table 1**). Importantly, there was no statically significant difference in adverse events.[2]

Additionally, omalizumab has been studied in patients receiving allergen immunotherapy (AIT). This is based on the argument that neutralization of IgE and reduced IgE receptor expression on mast cells and basophils should either eliminate or greatly reduce the severity of AIT-associated allergic reactions, including anaphylaxis. Omalizumab significantly improved the redness and swelling at immunotherapy injection sites and improved daily allergy severity scores.[2] Efficacy in preventing anaphylaxis was specifically studied using a rush AIT protocol. Rush immunotherapy is a process

Table 1 Meta-analysis of randomized controlled of omalizumab in allergic rhinitis		
Parameter	SMD/RR	P Value
Daily nasal symptom score	−0.443 (SMD)	P<.001
Daily ocular symptom score	−0.385 (SMD)	P<.001
Daily nasal medication symptom score	−0.421 (SMD)	P<.001
Proportion of days with emergency drug use	0.418 (RR)	P<.005
Rhinoconjunctivitis-specific QOL questionnaires	−0.286 (SMD)	P<.001
Overall evaluation	1.435 (RR)	P<.001

Abbreviations: QOL, quality of life; RR, relative risk; SMD, standardized mean difference.

in which patients serially receive AIT injections, typically in a single day, to rapidly achieve maintenance concentrations. Although often useful, rush immunotherapy is associated with a high risk for local and systemic allergic reactions. Casale and colleagues[3] found that omalizumab pretreatment reduced the adverse events associated with AIT and significantly reduced anaphylaxis (odds ratio, 0.17; $P = .026$). This result argues that similar results could be achieved with conventional AIT when used for treatment of AR (and asthma).

None of the other T2-targeting biologics have been specifically studied in AR. A handful of studies have assessed the efficacy of other T2-targeting biologics for the treatment of AR in the setting of comorbid asthma. Dupilumab (discussed in more detail later) is an anti-IL-4 receptor α (IL-4Rα) antibody that when dosed at 300 mg every 2 weeks was shown by Weinstein and colleagues[4] to significantly reduce AR-associated symptoms in patients with comorbid asthma. Only a nonstatistically significant trend was observed at the 200-mg dosing. Of note, no differences in asthma control were seen in subjects treated with either dose of dupilumab if they lacked comorbid perennial AR.[4]

No compelling studies of the IL-5/IL-5R-targeting biologics have been performed in AR. Although AR is often viewed in an oversimplified fashion as a purely IgE/mast cell–mediated disease, AR is strongly associated with the influx of eosinophils and attenuation of this eosinophilia underlies much of the efficacy of corticosteroids. As such, there is an argument for expecting efficacy from IL-5/IL-5R-targeting therapies in AR. In one study, although no specific analysis of nasal symptoms was reported, mepolizumab (humanized anti-IL-5 antibody) significantly reduced not only asthma exacerbations but also improved quality of life assessments in patients with severe asthma and self-reported upper airway disease.[5]

CHRONIC RHINOSINUSITIS WITHOUT NASAL POLYPS

Although extensively studied in CRS with NP (CRSwNPs) the efficacy of biologics in CRS without NPs (CRSsNP) is unexplored and remains theoretical. The failure to study biologics in CRSsNPs is largely based on the somewhat specious dogma that views CRSwNPs exclusively as a T2 inflammatory (IL-4^{high}/IL-5^{high}/IL-13^{high}) disease in contrast to CRSsNPs, which is typically viewed as a type 1 (interferon-γ^{high}) and/or type 3 (IL-17^{high}) disease.[6] As a consequence, CRSsNPs has typically not been considered an appropriate focus for T2-targeting biologics. Current studies provide compelling evidence against this oversimplified view of these conditions. For example, in a European study of CRSwNPs only 62% of NPs demonstrated only the T2 cytokine IL-5, an additional 23% were combinations of T2 with type 1 (interferon-γ) and/or type

3 (IL-17) cytokines, and fully 15% had no IL-5.[7] Similarly, in a North American study the identical 62% of CRSwNPs patients were shown to have isolated T2 disease.[8] The converse is true for CRS in the absence of NPs. Thus, in this European study[7] 20% of subjects had isolated T2 disease with an additional 3% displaying mixed T2 patterns and in the North American study fully 34% had isolated T2 disease.[8] Thus, arguably up to 38% of CRSwNP may be variably refractory to pure T2 targeting biologics and a similar proportion of CRSsNP patients (20%–34%) are currently being denied these agents, which are likely to be effective.

The investigation of T2-targeting biologics in CRSsNPs requires identification and validation of biomarkers to predict those who are likely to respond as the basis for investigation. Although some of these responsive patients are likely to have concomitant asthma or elevations in blood absolute eosinophil counts, such parameters are likely to greatly underidentify the potentially responsive population.[9] One of the best predictors of asthma responsiveness to biologics has been the identification of evidence for airway eosinophils, such as in induced sputum samples. Because functional endoscopic sinus surgery (FESS) is the mainstay of CRS therapy, a readily feasible approach to phenotyping CRSsNPs disease and predicting responsiveness to biologics is likely to have pathologic tissue samples analyzed for eosinophil content. Given the cost of biologics it may similarly be reasonable to avoid their use in patients with CRSsNP who have no evidence of eosinophilia on FESS-obtained tissue samples.

BIOLOGICS FOR NASAL POLYPOSIS
Omalizumab

The concept that targeting IgE may be efficacious in the treatment of NPs is based on the high tissue expression of IgE in these disorders including as active secretion by B cells and plasma cells and as surface IgE on mast cells.[10,11] This tissue expression of IgE correlates with the severity of the disease and rapidity of postsurgical polyp recurrence. The target of this IgE is unclear because tissue IgE concentrations do not correlate with the presence of atopy and, indeed, a high proportion of these patients are not atopic.[12] One target of the IgE has been proposed to be directed against antigens derived from pathogens present in CRSwNP including Staphylococcus aureus[13,14] and others.[15] One of first randomized, controlled study of omalizumab for NPs in 2013 involved a 16-week trial with 16 patents on active treatment versus eight on placebo.[16] Omalizumab treatment was associated with a significantly lower total nasal endoscopic score. Importantly, presence of aeroallergen sensitization did not influence outcome. In 2016, Nsouli and colleagues[17] conducted a 6-month trial involving nine subjects with NPs and asthma. In this small study, the omalizumab cohort (n = 5) demonstrated a 51% improvement in nasal endoscopic polyp scores (P<.001) and a 25% improvement in nasal function (P<.001). In a 2018 study, Bidder and colleagues[18] evaluated upper airway efficacy of omalizumab in a cohort of patients with severe asthma with coexistent CRSwNP. In this 16-week study, efficacy in improving the sinonasal outcome test (SNOT-22) was compared between 13 subjects who received omalizumab and 24 subjects treated with FESS and demonstrated similar improvements in both cohorts. Recently, two identical phase 3 clinical trials have been completed (Polyp 1/2) and their efficacy has recently been reported.[19] In these randomized controlled trials involving a total of 265 subjects, omalizumab demonstrated compelling evidence for efficacy including significant improvement in primary end points of change in average nasal congestion score and in endoscopically ascertained nasal polyp scores at 24 weeks (**Table 2**).

Table 2
Omalizumab efficacy in nasal polyposis

Parameter	Mean Change (Polyp 1/Polyp 2 Study[a])	P Value (Polyp 1/Polyp 2 Study)
Nasal congestion score	−0.89/−0.70	.0004/0.0017
Nasal polyp score	−1.08/−0.90	<.0001/0.014
SNOT-22 (0–110)	−24.70/−21.59	<.0001/<0.0001
Sense of smell score (0–3)	−0.56/−0.58	.0161/0.0024
Total nasal symptom score (0–12)	−2.97/−2.53	.0001/<0.0001
UPSIT smell assessment (0–40)	4.44/4.31	.0024/0.0011

Abbreviations: SNOT, sinonasal outcome test; UPSIT, University of Pennsylvania Smell Identification Test.
[a] Polyp 1 study, n = 138; Polyp 2 study, n = 127.

Interleukin-5 and Interleukin-5 Receptor–Targeting Therapies: Mepolizumab/Reslizumab/Benralizumab

IL-5 is a key cytokine for the stimulation, maturation, and survival of eosinophils. Elevated tissue eosinophilia and IL-5 levels are present in most patients with CRSwNP, making anti-IL5/IL-5R therapy an attractive potential treatment.

Mepolizumab

Mepolizumab is a humanized monoclonal antibody toward IL-5, which has shown promise in several studies related to CRSwNP. In a double-blind placebo-controlled study, patients with corticosteroid-refractory NP (n = 20) after treatment with mepolizumab demonstrated a reduction in total polyp score by 1.3 ± 1.72 versus 0.0 ± 0.94 in the placebo group (P = .028).[20] This study also demonstrated a trend toward improvement in symptom scores for smell, congestion, and posterior pharyngeal drainage. An additional double-blind randomized study showed that treatment with mepolizumab reduced the need for surgery in patients with severe recurrent bilateral NP. After treatment (n = 54), 30% of patients no longer met criteria for surgery based on endoscopic polyp scores and symptom severity scoring, compared with only 10% of the placebo group (n = 51; P = .006).[21] Additionally, in this same study patients treated with mepolizumab had significant reductions in SNOT-22 scores (−24.4; n = 32) when compared with placebo (−9.1; n = 42; P = .005). Another study investigating mepolizumab use in severe eosinophilic asthma demonstrated improvement in SNOT-22 scoring in patients with (−13.7; n = 44) and without (−8.6; n = 160) NP at baseline after treatment with mepolizumab compared with placebo control subjects (−1.9 [n = 34] and −3.7 [n = 167], respectively).[22]

Reslizumab

Reslizumab is also a humanized monoclonal antibody toward IL-5. In a small randomized controlled trial, 24 patients with bilateral NP received single doses of placebo or reslizumab at 1 or 3 mg/kg. Patients were noted to have improvement in total nasal polyp scores within 4 to 8 weeks, although the study was not sufficiently powered to determine significance.[23] At present, no other studies of this agent have been reported in regards to sinonasal outcome measures, although efficacy may be predicted based on the high expression of IL-5 in NPs and efficacy of other IL-5-targeting agents.

Benralizumab

Benralizumab is a humanized monoclonal antibody toward the specific receptor subunit for IL-5, IL-5Rα, and it is FDA approved for the treatment of severe eosinophilic asthma. It is being actively investigated for the treatment of CRSwNP but no efficacy studies have been reported. Two randomized double-blind placebo-controlled phase 3 clinical trials investigating benralizumab treatment of severe asthma underwent pooled subgroup analysis regarding NP. These studies demonstrated that the presence of NP was an independent predictor of enhanced efficacy of benralizumab treatment of severe asthma, separate from baseline peripheral blood eosinophilia.[24] Unfortunately, although NPs predicted greater efficacy for asthma, neither of these studies presented data for benralizumab for CRS or NP outcomes, although these observations invite further exploration.

Dupilumab

IL-4 and IL-13 are two key cytokines involved in the formation of nasal polyps in CRS. IL-4 promotes the terminal differentiation of naive T (Th0) cells into Th2 cells, promotes their survival, and thereby strongly enhances the presence of a T2^{high} state. IL-4 also contributes to mast cell activation. In contrast, IL-13 contributes to eosinophil migration, goblet cell metaplasia, mucus gland hyperplasia, and mucus hypersecretion. As a result of these mechanisms and numerous others, together these two cytokines drive processes central to tissue remodeling and NP formation in CRS. Dupilumab, as previously noted, is an anti-IL-4Rα antibody and, because this subunit is used by the IL-4 and IL-13 receptors, the engagement of dupilumab blocks the activities of both cytokines. Dupilumab was initially approved for moderate to severe atopic dermatitis in 2017, and was later approved for moderate to severe asthma in 2018.

In 2019, dupilumab was FDA approved for CRSwNP as a result of two pivotal trials evaluating its use for CRSwNP when compared with intranasal steroids.[25] Coprimary end points included a reduction in nasal polyp score and improved nasal obstruction or congestion scores. Significant improvements were observed in nasal polyp and congestion scores and in other measures of symptoms (total symptom score and SNOT-22). Dupilumab was also associated with remarkable improvements in olfaction and also in sinus severity as assessed by radiographic assessment (Lund-Mackay CT score) (**Table 3**). As a result of these findings, dupilumab became the first biologic treatment FDA approved for CRSwNP and can now be offered to patients failing conventional therapy.

Table 3
Dupilumab efficacy in nasal polyposis

Parameter	Least Squared Mean Change from Baseline (SINUS-24/SINUS-52 Trial[a])	P Value (SINUS-24/SINUS-52 Trial)
Nasal polyp score (0–8)	−2.06/−1.80	<.0001/<0.0001
Nasal congestion or obstruction score (0–3)	−0.89/−0.87	<.0001/<0.0001
Lund-Mackay CT score (0–24)	−7.44/−5.13	<.0001/<0.0001
Total symptom score (0–9)	−2.61/−2.44	<.0001/<0.0001
UPSIT smell assessment (0–40)	10.56/10.52	<.0001/<0.0001
Loss of smell score (0–3)	−1.12/−0.98	<.0001/<0.0001
SNOT-22 (0–110)	−21.12/−17.36	<.0001/<0.0001

[a] SINUS-24 study, n = 276; SINUS-52 study, n = 448.

SUMMARY

AR, most presentations of NP, and many presentations of CRS are T2^{high} inflammatory diseases of the upper airway characterized by expression of the interleukins IL-4, IL-5, and IL-13 and infiltration with an allergic inflammatory state with eosinophils, mast cells, basophils, and many other inflammatory cells. AR is mediated in large part by IgE directed against aeroallergens. Strong evidence exists for a role for IgE in contributing to the presence and severity of CRSwNPs, although the target of this IgE is less clear and may not involve aeroallergens. Given the immune basis for these conditions a strong theoretic basis exists for targeting these conditions with biologics that neutralize IgE (omalizumab), IL-5 (mepolizumab, reslizumab), the IL-5 receptor (benralizumab), or both IL-4 and IL-13 (dupilumab). For many of these agents, compelling clinical studies support their use in AR or NP and, indeed, one of these biologics (dupilumab) has recently received FDA approval for use in NPs. However, these agents are extremely expensive especially when considering the chronicity of these conditions and the likelihood that life-long therapy may prove warranted. Current therapies include combinations of medical therapies with nasal saline irrigation, antibiotics as appropriate, and combinations of topical and systemic corticosteroids. In many cases these approaches can provide long-term benefit and all, including surgery, are profoundly less expensive than biologics. Thus, future studies are imperative to address the cost effectiveness of biologics in these disorders, weighing in the adverse impact of these conditions on quality of life and determining their proper placement in therapy.

CLINICS CARE POINTS

- AR is mediated in large part by IgE and responds to IgE-targeting biologics (omalizumab).
- Efficacy of biologics in CRSsNPs is theoretically plausible but no efficacy studies have been performed.
- Biologics that target IgE, IL-5/IL-5 receptors, and the IL-4 receptor have all demonstrated efficacy in the treatment of NP.
- Currently dupilumab is the only biologic having FDA approval for the treatment of NPs.
- Future studies are essential to evaluate the cost effectiveness of biologics in the treatment of these disorders and their proper placement in therapy in comparison with medical and surgical therapies.

DISCLOSURE

L. Borish reports investigator-initiated research grants with Genentech, GSK, and Regeneron (all funds are awarded to the University of Virginia). L. Borish serves on an advisory board for Sanofi/Genzyme. W. Eschenbacher, M. Straesser, A. Knoeddler, and R.-C. Li have nothing to disclose.

REFERENCES

1. Chang TW. The pharmacological basis of anti-IgE therapy. Nat Biotechnol 2000; 18:157–62.

2. Yu C, Wang K, Cui X, et al. Clinical efficacy and safety of omalizumab in the treatment of allergic rhinitis: a systematic review and meta-analysis of randomized clinical trials. Am J Rhinol Allergy 2019;34(2):196–208.

3. Casale TB, Busse WW, Kline JN, et al. Omalizumab pretreatment decreases acute reactions after rush immunotherapy for ragweed-induced seasonal allergic rhinitis. J Allergy Clin Immunol 2006;117:134–40.
4. Weinstein SF, Katial R, Jayawardena S, et al. Efficacy and safety of dupilumab in perennial allergic rhinitis and comorbid asthma. J Allergy Clin Immunol 2018;142: 171–177 e1.
5. Prazma CM, Albers F, Mallett S, et al. Mepolizumab improves patient outcomes and reduces exacerbations in severe asthma patients with comorbid upper airway disease. American Academy of Asthma, Allergy, and Immunology National Meeting, San Francisco, February 22 - February 26, 2019.
6. Meltzer EO, Hamilos DL, Hadley JA, et al. Rhinosinusitis: establishing definitions for clinical research and patient care. J Allergy Clin Immunol 2004;114:155–212.
7. Wang X, Zhang N, Bo M, et al. Diversity of TH cytokine profiles in patients with chronic rhinosinusitis: a multicenter study in Europe, Asia, and Oceania. J Allergy Clin Immunol 2016;138:1344–53.
8. Stevens WW, Peters AT, Tan BK, et al. Associations between inflammatory endotypes and clinical presentations in chronic rhinosinusitis. J Allergy Clin Immunol Pract 2019;7:2812–28120 e3.
9. Steinke JW, Smith AR, Carpenter DJ, et al. Lack of efficacy of symptoms and medical history in distinguishing the degree of eosinophilia in nasal polyps. J Allergy Clin Immunol Pract 2017;5:1582–8.e3.
10. Bachert C, Gevaert P, Holtappels G, et al. Total and specific IgE in nasal polyps is related to local eosinophilic inflammation. J Allergy Clin Immunol 2001;107: 607–14.
11. Baba S, Kondo K, Suzukawa M, et al. Distribution, subtype population, and IgE positivity of mast cells in chronic rhinosinusitis with nasal polyps. Ann Allergy Asthma Immunol 2017;119:120–8.
12. Johns CB, Laidlaw TM. Elevated total serum IgE in nonatopic patients with aspirin-exacerbated respiratory disease. Am J Rhinol Allergy 2014;28:287–9.
13. Van Zele T, Gevaert P, Watelet JB, et al. Staphylococcus aureus colonization and IgE antibody formation to enterotoxins is increased in nasal polyposis. J Allergy Clin Immunol 2004;114:981–3.
14. Huvenne W, Hellings PW, Bachert C. Role of staphylococcal superantigens in airway disease. Int Arch Allergy Immunol 2013;161:304–14.
15. Takeda K, Sakakibara S, Yamashita K, et al. Allergic conversion of protective mucosal immunity against nasal bacteria in patients with chronic rhinosinusitis with nasal polyposis. J Allergy Clin Immunol 2019;143:1163–1175 e15.
16. Gevaert P, Calus L, Van Zele T, et al. Omalizumab is effective in allergic and nonallergic patients with nasal polyps and asthma. J Allergy Clin Immunol 2013;131:110–116 e1.
17. Nsouli TM, Bellanti JA, Diliberto NZ, et al. Is there a role for recombinant antiimmunoglobulin E therapy in the management of nasal polyposis? Ann Allergy Asthma Immunol 2015;115(Suppl. 1):A117.
18. Bidder T, Sahota J, Rennie C, et al. Omalizumab treats chronic rhinosinusitis with nasal polyps and asthma together: a real life study. Rhinology 2018;56:42–5.
19. Gevaert P, Bachert C, Corren J, et al. Omalizumab efficacy and safety in nasal polyposis: results from two parallel, double-blind, placebo-controlled trials. Ann Allergy Asthma Immunol 2019;123:S17.
20. Gevaert P, Van Bruaene N, Cattaert T, et al. Mepolizumab, a humanized anti-IL-5 mAb, as a treatment option for severe nasal polyposis. J Allergy Clin Immunol 2011;128:989–95.e1-8.

21. Bachert C, Sousa AR, Lund VJ, et al. Reduced need for surgery in severe nasal polyposis with mepolizumab: randomized trial. J Allergy Clin Immunol 2017;140: 1024–31.e14.
22. Chupp GL, Bradford ES, Albers FC, et al. Efficacy of mepolizumab add-on therapy on health-related quality of life and markers of asthma control in severe eosinophilic asthma (MUSCA): a randomised, double-blind, placebo-controlled, parallel-group, multicentre, phase 3b trial. Lancet Respir Med 2017;5:390–400.
23. Gevaert P, Lang-Loidolt D, Lackner A, et al. Nasal IL-5 levels determine the response to anti-IL-5 treatment in patients with nasal polyps. J Allergy Clin Immunol 2006;118:1133–41.
24. Harrison T, Werkstrom V, Wu Y, et al. Clinical efficacy of benralizumab in patients with severe uncontrolled eosinophilic asthma and nasal polyposis: pooled analysis of the SIROCCO and CALIMA trials. J Allergy Clin Immunol 2018;141:AB12.
25. Bachert C, Han JK, Desrosiers M, et al. Efficacy and safety of dupilumab in patients with severe chronic rhinosinusitis with nasal polyps (LIBERTY NP SINUS-24 and LIBERTY NP SINUS-52): results from two multicentre, randomised, double-blind, placebo-controlled, parallel-group phase 3 trials. Lancet 2019;394: 1638–50.

Biologics for the Treatments of Allergic Conditions
Severe Asthma

Marco Caminati, MD[a],*, Diego Bagnasco, MD[b],
Lanny J. Rosenwasser, MD[c],[1], Andrea Vianello, MD[d],[e],
Gianenrico Senna, MD[f]

KEYWORDS

- Severe asthma • Anti IL-33 • Benralizumab • Dupilumab • Mepolizumab
- Omalizumab • Reslizumab • Tezepelumab

KEY POINTS

- Currently marketed biologics for severe asthma provide a revolutionary treatment option by selectively targeting specific steps of the immune inflammation cascade within the Th2 high patterns.
- Upcoming molecules are able to address epithelial and innate immunity potentially allowing to a better management of severe asthma beyond Th2 high phenotypes.
- A permanent disease-modifying effect of biologics is not yet completely clear so that optimal treatment duration, the possibility of a dose treatment modulation, the place and relevance of ICS in best responders still represent controversial aspects.
- Long-term safety, especially when interacting with epithelial and innate immunity needs to be further investigated and should be carefully evaluated in patient selection.
- Both basic research and real-word evidence are needed to address the open challenges and unmet needs.

Funded by: CRUI2020.
[a] Department of Medicine, Allergy and Clinical Immunology Section, University of Verona and Verona University Hospital, Piazzale Scuro 10, Verona 37134, Italy; [b] Allergy and Respiratory Diseases, IRCCS Policlinico San Martino, University of Genoa, Largo Rosanna Benzi, 10, Genoa 16132, Italy; [c] UMKC School of Medicine, Kansas City, MO, USA; [d] Respiratory Pathophysiology Division, University of Padua, Padua, Italy; [e] Dipartimento di Scienze CardioToraco Vascolari e Sanità Pubblica, Via Nicolo' Giustiniani, 2, Padua 35128, Italy; [f] Department of Medicine, Allergy and Clinical Immunology School, University of Verona & Asthma Center and Allergy Unit, Verona University Hospital, Piazzale Scuro 10, Verona 37134, Italy
[1] Present address: 14129 Nicklaus Drive, Overland Park, KS 66223.
* Corresponding author. Department of Medicine, University of Verona and Verona University Hospital, Piazzale Scuro 10, Verona 37134, Italy. ;
E-mail address: marco.caminati@univr.it

INTRODUCTION

Patients with asthma requiring a second controller and/or systemic corticosteroids for a satisfactory disease control, although regularly treated with high-dose inhaled corticosteroids, are affected by severe asthma. Similarly, patients whose disease remains uncontrolled despite the previously mentioned pharmacologic strategies are defined as having severe asthma. This definition comes from the recent International European Respiratory Society/ American Thoracic Society (ERS/ATS) guidelines.[1,2] According to the Global Initiative for Asthma (GINA) international recommendations, daytime symptoms (more than twice a week), night-time symptoms, activity limitation, and the need for rescue medication more than twice a week represent the hallmarks of poor asthma control. In particular, if at least 3 of the previously mentioned conditions occur, the patient is experiencing uncontrolled asthma.[3]

The prevalence of severe asthma lacks of univocal estimation, ranging from 1.8% to 38% in different studies.[4-6] Differences in terms of population samples, definitions, and methodology characterizing the published reports may account for that variability. On the other hand, severe asthma, in particular when difficult to control, is undoubtedly responsible for the major burden of the disease in terms of both social and economic implications. In fact, major asthma exacerbations, asthma-related emergency room admissions, hospitalizations, and overall quality-of-life impairment are typical features of the severe phenotype in comparison with the mild or moderate ones.[4,7] The known complex cross-talking between genetic heterogeneity and environmental triggers, and the relevance of difficult to manage comorbidities may provide an explanation to severe asthma burden despite the variety and quality of traditional treatment options. In fact, severe asthma management still represents a major challenge for clinicians and affected patients.[1,8]

Biologic drugs are determining a true revolution in the field. Recently marketed, they are able to selectively target one or more molecular players by blocking their effect within the inflammation cascade.[9] The currently available biologics are mostly active on Th2/eosinophilic phenotype molecules.[10] The so-called Th2 high inflammatory pattern characterizes most patients affected by severe asthma; however, ongoing pharmacologic and clinical research is exploring new treatment options able to interact with Th2 low phenotypes, although regarding a smaller proportion of patients, but still difficult to treat due to reduced response to inhaled corticosteroids (ICS) and oral corticosteroids (OCS).[2]

Currently placed as an add on therapy for patients not satisfactory controlled by GINA step 5 treatment options, biologics provide a unique opportunity to improve the quality of life of patients with severe asthma by definitely achieving disease control and reducing/stopping their oral steroid dependence.[2,3] Under a wider perspective, the use of biologics allows to contain indirect costs and the socio-economic burden of severe asthma.

The present work aims at providing an overview of the evidence on immunologic and clinical effects of biologic drugs, including a focus on the current unmet needs in the field.

A PubMed and Medline search was performed. The following keywords were selected: severe asthma, dupilumab, omalizumab, reslizumab, mepolizumab, benralizumab, tezepelumab, immunology of severe asthma. Papers published up to Dec 2019 were considered. Original articles, randomized clinical trials, and review papers relevant to the topic were evaluated for inclusion in the review.

BIOLOGICS FOR SEVERE ASTHMA: WHAT'S ON
Omalizumab

Mechanism
Omalizumab is a humanized monoclonal antibody, able to bind the site for high affinity of immunoglobulin (Ig)E receptor, leading to blocking interaction of the Ig with FcεRI located on mast cells, antigen-presenting cells, and basophils.[11–13] The action on these cells reduces the production of type 2 cytokines and T2 inflammation.[14] Studies carried out on omalizumab have also shown that this drug is able, through an action on IgE carrier B cells, to cause a state of anergy causing a reduction/suspension of the response to antigenic/allergenic stimulation[15] (**Fig. 1**).

Target patients
Omalizumab has shown the best performance in adult and pediatric patients, with moderate-to-severe persistent asthma that a skin or in vitro positive perennial aeroallergen, whose symptoms are not adequately controlled by maximal inhalation therapy[16] and with total IgE 30 to 700 IU/mL in those ages 12 and older and IgE 30 to 1300 IU/mL in those ages 6 to 11. The combined elevation of exhaled nitric oxide (FeNO) ($\geq$19.5 parts per billion), peripheral blood eosinophils ($\geq$260 per microliter), and periostin ($\geq$50 ng/mL) was reported as a predictor of better response.[17] However, according to more recent evidence, omalizumab efficacy is independent of the baseline blood eosinophilia.[18,19]

Major outcomes
The marketed formulation is a subcutaneous injection at the dose of 0.016 mg/IgE in IU/mL × body weight in kilograms. Omalizumab has been extensively studied, both in clinical trials and in real life and has demonstrated excellent efficacy in reducing asthma exacerbations and the use of systemic corticosteroids in treated patients.[20] As happens also for all biological drugs in asthma, the efficacy of omalizumab is better in well-selected patients. Omalizumab was first marketed in 2003, when the US Food and Drug Administration approved the use of this molecule in the United States.[16]

From the analysis of 12 trials, for a total of 6427 patients, it was observed that the therapy, if used in addition to the ICS/long-acting beta2 agonists (LABA) combination, reduced the risk of exacerbations at the end of the study (relative risk, RR = 0.57) and the need for systemic corticosteroid therapy (RR 1.80, 95% confidence interval [CI] = 1.42–2.28).[16,21] Similar promising results were also observed in improving quality of life, as measured by the Asthma Quality of Life Questionnaire, which is higher in patients treated with omalizumab than in control patients (0.33; 95% CI 0.27–0.38), but still lower than the minimally clinically important difference of 0.5.[22] Similar efficacy could be observed in lung function tests.[16] Therefore considering the clinical data from the randomized controlled trials, the clinician should focus on reducing systemic steroid use and exacerbations in patients treated with omalizumab, and to a lesser extent on the variation of the quality of life and respiratory function questionnaires, both results not always varied by therapy.

Mepolizumab

Mechanism
Mepolizumab is a humanized murine IgG1k monoclonal antibody. By selectively targeting the α-chain of interleukin (IL)-5 it prevents its binding to IL-5 receptor α (IL-5Rα), which is expressed on the surface of eosinophils and basophils.[23] As a consequence, eosinophil differentiation, activation, and growth are inactivated[23] (see **Fig. 1**). Of note, the reported 70% block of eosinophil maturation in the bone marrow,

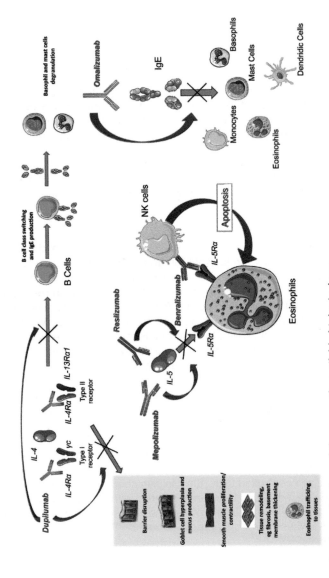

Fig. 1. Overview of main mechanisms of the currently available biologic drugs.

including a partial but significant depletion of eosinophil myelocytes and metamyelocytes, has been described when a dose of 750 mg was administered intravenously.[24] On the opposite, the marketed dosing regimen did not show to impact on eosinophil progenitors in the blood or bone marrow while a restart of physiologic eosinophil maturation has been detected approximately 3 months after mepolizumab discontinuation. It may account for the fast airway inflammation and asthma symptoms relapse.[24–26] Concerning bronchial district, a dose-dependent but still partial (and not significant with mepolizumab 100 mg)[24] eosinophil depletion has been observed.[25,27] Of note, IL-5 cannot be considered the only cytokine regulating the eosinophil bronchial homing; in fact other molecules including eotaxin, which are not targeted by mepolizumab, may play a relevant role.[9,25]

Target patients

Blood eosinophil count ≥300 cells/μL has been identified as the minimum requirement for the best response to mepolizumab within the population with severe asthma.[23,27] Higher eosinophil count may predict even better response regarding specific parameters. A post hoc analysis of DREAM and MENSA trials highlighted that the lung function increase was more evident for patients with baseline eosinophil counts ≥500 cells/μL.[28] Also, the exacerbation rate reduction was greater in patients with 3 or ≥4 (but not in that with 2) exacerbations in the previous year.[27]

On the opposite, body mass index did not result to be a covariate for exacerbation rate in the analysis of the DREAM trial.[27] The presence of nasal polyps does not seem to affect mepolizumab benefit on asthma, although the drug effect on that comorbidity is controversial.[29,30]

Major outcomes

The approved dose of mepolizumab is 100 mg every 4 weeks. The major clinical outcomes demonstrated by the published trials and subsequent analyses include asthma exacerbations and systemic glucocorticoid.[31] A 30% to 50% reduction in number of exacerbations and a 50% decrease of oral steroid (OCS) dose (odds ratio 2.39 for mepolizumab vs placebo [95% CI 1.25–4.56; P = .008]), were overall described in treated patients.[32,33] More in detail, SIRIUS trial reported a 90% to 100% OCS reduction in 23% of patients and a 75% to less than 90% OCS reduction in 17%. In 36% of active group (vs 56% of placebo group) no OCS change was observed.[32]

A significant improvement of lung function, more consistent in patients with baseline eosinophil counts ≥500 cells/μL, was shown by most of studies.[28,33,34]

Reslizumab

Mechanism

Reslizumab is a recombinant humanized IgG4k monoclonal antibody able to block IL-5 and interfere with its functions.[10] Its mechanism of action is similar to mepolizumab (see **Fig. 1**). The only substantial difference with mepolizumab is regarding the intravenous way of administration. Tailoring the dose through a weight-adjusted approach seems to provide an additional opportunity and a more robust pharmacologic effect according to some evidence[35]; a further reduction of airways eosinophilia (sputum eosinophilia), in comparison with mepolizumab, has been described; however the topic is under debate.[36]

Target patients

Blood eosinophil count ≥400 cells/μL and 12% forced expiratory volume in 1 second (FEV1) reversibility characterize the best responders to reslizumab among patients with severe asthma.[37] The coexistence of (self-reported) chronic sinusitis with nasal polyposis (CSwNP) seems to enhance reslizumab effect on asthma control.

Major outcomes

Reslizumab is approved at the dosage of 3 mg/kg every 4 weeks. It demonstrated to determine a 50% to 59% reduction of the annual exacerbation rate when compared with placebo.[37] The same effect rises to 83% in patients with CSwNP and higher blood eosinophilia level (400 cells/μL). A significant increase in time to first exacerbation and in the number of patients with a year free of exacerbations has also been described,[38] together with pre-bronchodilator FEV1 improvement. Reslizumab was also responsible for a 70% to 50% decrease in OCS daily dose.

Benralizumab

Mechanism

Benralizumab, a fully humanized afucosylated IgG1κ monoclonal antibody, selectively binds an IL-5 receptor α (IL-5Rα) epitope and interferes with IL-5 signaling, independently of the ligand presence.[39] IL-5 Rα is restrictedly expressed on eosinophils and basophils, but also on their progenitors in the bone marrow, thus it provides the right target for selective cell depletion.[40] Benralizumab depletes IL-5Rα-expressing cells through a second way, that is an antibody-directed cell-mediated cytotoxicity (see **Fig. 1**). The previously mentioned afucosylation of the monoclonal antibody oligosaccharide core significantly enhances the affinity to human Fcγ receptor IIIa (FcγRIIIa), mainly expressed on natural killer (NK) cells. When activated by interaction with benralizumab, NK cells contribute to a robust depletion of eosinophils in the bone marrow and blood, and to an almost complete depletion in sputum and tissues.[39] No evidence of a similar effect, which seems to sustain a more consistent clinical effect,[39] is currently available for other anti–IL-5 drugs.

Target patients

Benralizumab has demonstrated the greatest effect in patients with severe asthma and blood eosinophils $\geq$300 cells/μL.[41] A pooled analysis of the SIROCCO and CALIMA studies looked for predictors of enhanced response to benralizumab.[42] Besides peripheral eosinophils, OCS dependence, the presence of nasal polyposis, and forced vital capacity less than 65% of predicted were identified as relevant parameters. More precisely, according to a similar post hoc analysis,[43] patients combining at baseline high blood eosinophils and a history of 3 or more exacerbations in the previous year experienced a more robust reduction of annual exacerbation rate during the treatment course. In addition, the coexistence of obesity or fixed airflow obstruction before the treatment start did not hamper the positive impact of benralizumab on lung function.[41]

Major outcomes

The recommended dose of benralizumab is 30 mg every 4 weeks for the first 3 doses, and then every 8 weeks.[41] In patients with $\geq$300 blood eosinophils/μL, 3 main clinical outcomes were reported and confirmed by different studies: (1) asthma exacerbation rate. According to SIROCCO and CALIMA trials,[44,45] benralizumab reduced asthma exacerbations by approximately 50% and 36% (28% for the every 8-week dosing arm), respectively. (2) Oral steroid intake. A median OCS reduction 75%, versus 25% in the placebo group was observed during the treatment (P<.001).[46] (3) Lung function. A clinically significant improvement of pre-bronchodilator FEV1 was reported by the BISE study. The change was greater than 80 mL (95% CI 0–150; P = .04) after 3 months of therapy.[47]

Of note, due to its peculiar mechanism, benralizumab action is independent of IL-5 levels, which can increase during asthma exacerbation. It provides the rationale for treating acute asthma exacerbations with benralizumab as well, although little evidence is available on that at the moment.[48]

Dupilumab

Mechanism
Dupilumab is a fully humanized molecule able to bind, with high affinity and specifically, the α subunit of the IL-4 receptor, shared by the IL-4 type I receptor complex (IL-4α/γc) and IL-4/IL-13 type II receptor complex (IL-4α/IL-13Rα), and to inhibit the signal of both cytokines.[49] Therefore, due to the crucial role that these 2 cytokines play in type 2 inflammation, their inhibition is able to reduce/suppress the inflammatory response, the cytokine and chemokine cascade induced by their activity[49] (see **Fig. 1**).

Target patients
From the subanalysis carried out observing the characteristics of the patients enrolled in the registration studies, it was concluded that subjects with a more marked type 2 inflammation, characterized by high values of eosinophilia and exhaled nitric oxide (FeNO), are those who better respond to treatment with dupilumab.[50–52] In particular, a post hoc study of QUEST[50] showed that patients with eosinophils and FeNO values above 150 cell/μL and 25 ppb, respectively, had better benefits. On the other hand, in the VENTURE[52] study the biomarker statistics were not as clear-cut, with the exception of severe exacerbations, which can be influenced overall by the FeNO value (with better outcome in the case of FeNO$\geq$50 ppb or $\geq$25 to <50 ppb compared with <25 ppb). A possible cause of these differences between the 2 studies could be the use of OCS by patients in the VENTURE[52] study. Therefore studies show that dupilumab is able to modify the previously mentioned endpoints, statistically differently from placebo, in patients with blood eosinophilia less than 150 cell/μL or FeNO less than 25 ppb in QUEST[50] or in patients with less than 150 EOS/μL in VENTURE.[52]

Major outcomes
As with other biological drugs developed for asthma, the effects of the molecule on exacerbations of disease and reduction of systemic corticosteroid use were primarily assessed in dupilumab studies.

In the main randomized controlled trials, dupilumab (200 or 300 mg every 2 weeks) was shown to significantly reduce the annual exacerbation rate by almost 50% in 52 weeks in the QUEST study, where this outcome was placed as the primary endpoint,[50] data confirmed by even shorter 24-week studies (DRI12544)[51] and VENTURE.[52] The hospitalization/response rate was also found to be reduced by 46.8% in QUEST. In addition to the already mentioned reduction of exacerbations, dupilumab has proven to be able to save OCS in dependent patients in the VENTURE study.[52] In this study, dupilumab (300 mg every 2 weeks) made it possible to reduce the daily OCS dose significantly more than placebo at week 24 (end of OCS maintenance phase) with baseline (after OCS dosage optimization).

Further subanalysis showed that dupilumab was also able to reduce the steroid dose to <5 mg prednisone in more than 50% of cases.[52,53] Because it is a drug developed for a respiratory disease, pulmonary function, although not always as the primary outcome, has also been evaluated. Dupilumab was found to increase lung function in all studies, at both 200 and 300 mg every 2 weeks. The function values measured by FEV1 showed a significant increase after 12 and 24 weeks of treatment.[50,51] The same results were also observed after only 2 weeks of dupilumab therapy[52–54] (P<.001 vs placebo where reported[53,54]).

BIOLOGICS FOR SEVERE ASTHMA: THE NEAR FUTURE

The most recent advances in the field have suggested epithelial barrier dysfunction as the primum movens of asthma pathogenesis.[9] Besides anatomic integrity, mainly related to genetic predisposition and smoking habit, epithelial barrier efficiency relies on innate immunity competence. An impaired immunologic first-line response may trigger an unbalanced inflammation, meaning Th2 polarized response and altered tissue repair processes leading to airway remodeling and further epithelial physical inefficiency.[55]

In the light of that evidence, master cytokines regulating the cross talk between epithelial cells and innate/adaptive immunity have been identified as potential pharmacologic treatment targets. Among them, TSLP (thymic stromal lymphoprotein) and IL-33 are currently under investigation in clinical trials and will provide new therapeutic options in the near future.[9]

Tezepelumab

Mechanism
Tezepelumab is a humanized monoclonal antibody blocking TSLP by preventing the interaction with its receptor complex.[56] This cytokine expresses the innate immunity activation. Produced by the epithelium, it regulates dendritic cell functions, polarizes the differentiation of naive T cells into mature CD4 T cells, activates B cells, and regulates Th2 cytokine production (mainly IL-4, IL-5, IL-13). The last effect is also mediated by direct activation of ILC2 (innate lymphoid cells).[57]

Target patients
When considering tezepelumab mechanism of action, its efficacy on both Th-2 high and low asthma phenotypes is quite clear. In fact, when activated by allergens or environmental stimuli, including viruses and pollutants, it interferes with the impaired immune response before its evolution in a Type 2 high or Type 2 low pattern and regardless the individual atopic status.[9,56]

No specific markers of Th2 phenotype such as IgE or eosinophils were considered when selecting the study population of a recent phase 2b trial.[58] The study, the only one currently available, included adult patients with uncontrolled asthma (at least 2 exacerbations requiring systemic glucocorticoids in the previous year) despite medium-dose to high-dose inhaled glucocorticoid and long-acting β-agonist, FEV1 between 40% and 80% of predicted and at least a 12% and 200 mL improvement with bronchodilator.

Major outcomes
Exacerbation rate was 61%, 71%, and 66% lower than the placebo in the low-dose (70 mg subcutaneously every 4 weeks), medium-dose (210 mg subcutaneously every 4 weeks), and high-dose groups (280 mg subcutaneously every 2 weeks) respectively, regardless of initial eosinophil level. Also a significantly longer time to first exacerbation in patients receiving the medium-dose and high-dose tezepelumab versus placebo was observed, and all tezepelumab groups experienced a relevant pre-bronchodilator FEV1 increase versus placebo.[58]

Anti–Interleukin-33

IL-33 belongs to alarmins family and is produced by epithelial cells in response to the interactions with environmental triggers or inflammatory factors. Its activation depends on protease digestive process of its pro-cytokine form.[59] In view of its functions, IL-33 is believed to play a key role both in type 1 and type 2 inflammation. In fact it interacts with innate immunity, particularly dendritic cells and it is also able to initiate a type 2 immunity inflammatory cascade by polarizing Th2 cells and ILC2 cells.[60] Very recently, a phase 2 12-week proof-of-concept trial, that enrolled 296 adult patients with moderate-to-severe asthma who were not well controlled on LABA and ICS therapy, evaluated IL-33 as a therapeutic target in severe asthma.[61] REGN 3500, a humanized monoclonal antibody to all IL-33 molecules regardless of amino terminus, demonstrated its superiority versus placebo in significantly improving asthma control and lung function, with an optimal safety profile. The greatest effect was observed in patients with blood eosinophil levels $\geq$300 cells/μL. The potential use of anti–IL-33 antibody has not yet been evaluated by any regulatory authority, and an asthma clinical trial program is currently under development.[61]

REAL-LIFE PERSPECTIVE: RATIONALE AND MAJOR EVIDENCE

In parallel to the randomized controlled clinical trials, several real-life trials have been described. The importance of these evaluations also in real life is strategic for a better and greater understanding of the effects of a drug, otherwise studied only in selected patients. In fact, it is well known that patients in randomized clinical trials are usually younger, with better fitness and, above all, with fewer comorbidities than those who, once the drug is marketed, will use experimental drugs.[62,63] The importance of real-life studies is also revealed with regard to the duration of treatment. The timing of randomized controlled trials is in fact generally short, with a mean duration of 6 to 12 months, inadequate to assess the long-term effects of the drugs, those of withdrawal after long periods of treatment, and disease control after discontinuation of treatment.

Particularly, it has been observed that patients with severe asthma, treated in real life, are very different from those in clinical trials, both for omalizumab[20] and mepolizumab.[64] Because of its long-standing commercialization, omalizumab has long been studied not only in randomized controlled trials, but also in real life.[20,63] This type of study has made it possible to clarify and deepen what emerged in the trials regarding the safety, even after long periods of administration, the efficacy of the drug in patients with comorbidities and its impact on the latter.[20] Although there are unavoidable differences between the real-life population and randomized patients in the trials, with the former having a significantly lower FEV1 and a higher IgE level, the efficacy of the drug in symptom control, exacerbations and improvement of respiratory function is confirmed even after only 4 months of treatment.[65–67] As said, one of the aims of studies in RL is to assess what happens when therapy is discontinued, and consequently to seek an optimal duration of therapy. In this respect, the results for omalizumab are not entirely straightforward. In fact, the data in real life are limited; recently a study conducted on 49 patients showed a persistent effect of more than 4 years after OMA interruption, extended to 6 years in 60% of cases.[68]

Although mepolizumab has been developed and marketed, some data about real life are available. The efficacy in reducing exacerbations, OCS daily dose and steroid dependence has been demonstrated in a 1 year observational study performed on 138 patients.[69] Similar results were subsequently confirmed also in another observational trial performed on 61 patients with severe asthma.[70] The first study also described side effects of 12 months of administration, with few side effects and already well described in clinical trials, confirming a comforting safety profile.[69] Regarding safety profile, another study, on 143 patients, described only 6 discontinuations of the drug, 5 of them due to poor efficacy and only 1 because of the occurrence of adverse events (urticaria).[71] Real-life experience permitted also the observation of the effect of mepolizumab on patients previously treated with other biologic drugs, particularly omalizumab. Despite this has been performed in a clinical trial evaluating the effect of this therapeutic switch,[72] usually in trials the previous administration of another monoclonal antibody is an exclusion criteria for randomization, and for this reason the data from these patients is quite poor. In a 1-year observational study, performed on 27 patients previously treated with omalizumab and switched to mepolizumab due to poor efficacy of the anti-IgE drug, a significant reduction of exacerbations, OCS intake, improvement of FEV1 has been proven.[73] As for omalizumab, also mepolizumab has been investigated in real life for its effect on lung function. In a multicenter observational Italian study, involving 134 patients with severe asthma, the effect of the administration of anti–IL-5 drug for 6 months on lung function tests has been observed, with an increase of FEV1 of approximately 200 mL.[74]

Among the main objectives of research in severe asthma and in biologic therapies, there is the discovery of biomarkers able to predict the response to the drugs. In a subanalysis of the DREAM study,[27] Ortega and colleagues[28] described the relationship between the baseline eosinophil level before mepolizumab administration and the response to the drug. In a subanalysis of an Italian real-life study instead has not confirmed a similar trend.[75]

About reslizumab, a trial on 26 patients evidenced an efficacy of the drug in reducing exacerbations, glucocorticoid doses, and being also able to improve the control of the disease (measured with ACQ-6 questionnaire).[76] About benralizumab and dupilumab, due to their recent commercialization, only a few data about their efficacy in real life are available.

SUMMARY AND UNMET NEEDS

The opportunity to selectively interfere with specific steps of the immune inflammatory cascade and consequently achieve better or complete asthma control is something completely new in the field, and the revolution is still ongoing, including drugs under development and others very recently marketed.[9,10] Despite a relatively limited experience, robust evidence supports a strong safety and efficacy profile for each one of the available biologics. On the other hand, whether these molecules are able to provide a long-lasting disease-modifying effect independent of treatment continuation, and when it occurs, is still under debate.[9] For that reason, the optimal treatment duration, the possibility of a dose treatment modulation in high or poor responders, the place and relevance of ICS in best responders still represent controversial aspects. Among the everyday challenges clinicians using biologics have to face, the optimal patient selection represents a major one. In fact, low-nonresponders among patients matching prescription criteria and the theoretic best responder profile of that biologic are rather frequent, as well as subjects characterized by overlapping eligibility.[8,77] A number of biomarkers have been explored but up to now no one is able to specifically predict the response to one biologic drug.[78] The research is still ongoing; focusing on composite indexes, including patients' comorbidities, could improve patients' selection accuracy and more in general biologic therapy sustainability.

Management of the so-called Th2 low phenotypes represents another major challenge. In fact, although regarding a smaller proportion of patients with asthma, they are usually characterized by poor response to steroids, whether systemic or inhaled, and frequent exacerbations. The currently available biologics are not able to specifically address Th2 low phenotypes.[79] However, the upcoming molecules targeting epithelial-innate immunity besides beyond eosinophilic pattern, namely anti-TSLP and anti–IL-33, could provide an opportunity for some Th2 low phenotypes.

Most importantly, so far no one of the biologics currently in use have been related to major safety issues. In particular, eosinophil partial or complete depletion has not been related to any specific disease or dysregulation, in terms of infections, tumors, or auto-immune diseases, in animal models and human subjects.[10,31] Although the premarketing research and real-life evidence when available have provided for all of them an optimal safety profile, which is also conceptually supported by their extremely selective way of action, the long-term safety remains something to be carefully investigated in the real-life setting. With regard to some upcoming molecules, interfering with innate and epithelial immunity may raise potential issues and suggest a very careful patient selection especially when other immune-mediated diseases coexist. However, apart from speculative considerations, the currently available evidence cannot support any warning or specific recommendation on the topic.

In conclusion, biologics for severe asthma have substantially contributed to increase the standard of care, to reduce drug (particularly OCS)-related morbidity, and most importantly to ameliorate patients' quality of life.

Both basic research and real-word evidence are needed to address the open challenges and unmet needs.

CLINICS CARE POINTS

- Monoclonal antibodies targeting cytokines or their receptors within the severe asthma inflammation cascade are able allow to achieve better or complete asthma control and to significantly reduce or interrupt the use of systemic steroids.
- According to the evidence coming from clinical trials and real-life studies, biologic therapies for severe asthma provide an optimal safety and tolerability profile; however, the potential long-term effects need to be carefully monitored.
- Some practical aspects related to the management of biologic therapies for severe asthma remain under discussion: the optimal treatment duration, the possibility of a dose treatment modulation in high or poor responders, the place and relevance of ICS in best responders.
- The optimal candidate selection to each biologic treatment still remains challenging, especially in patients with overlapping eligibility. A number of biomarkers have been explored but up to now no one is able to specifically predict the response to one biologic drug.

DISCLOSURE

The authors have nothing to disclose.

REFERENCES

1. Chung KF, Wenzel SE, Brozek JL, et al. International ERS/ATS guidelines on definition, evaluation and treatment of severe asthma. Eur Respir J 2014;43:343–73.

2. Holguin F, Cardet JC, Chung KF, et al. Management of severe asthma: a European Respiratory Society/American Thoracic Society guideline. Eur Respir J 2020;55 [pii:1900588].

3. Global Initiative for Asthma. GINA, 2019. Available at: http://ginasthma.org/. Accessed December 23, 2019.

4. Chen S, Golam S, Myers J, et al. Systematic literature review of the clinical, humanistic, and economic burden associated with asthma uncontrolled by GINA Steps 4 or 5 treatment. Curr Med Res Opin 2018;34:2075–88.

5. Hekking PP, Wener RR, Amelink M, et al. The prevalence of severe refractory asthma. J Allergy Clin Immunol 2015;135:896–902.

6. Vianello A, Caminati M, Andretta M, et al. Prevalence of severe asthma according to the drug regulatory agency perspective: An Italian experience. World Allergy Organ J 2019;12:100032.

7. O'Neill S, Sweeney J, Patterson CC, et al. The cost of treating severe refractory asthma in the UK: an economic analysis from the British Thoracic Society Difficult Asthma Registry. Thorax 2015;70:376–8.

8. Caminati M, Senna G. Uncontrolled severe asthma: starting from the unmet needs. Curr Med Res Opin 2019;35:175–7.

9. Caminati M, Polk B, Rosenwasser LJ. What have recent advances in therapy taught us about severe asthma disease mechanisms? Expert Rev Clin Immunol 2019;15:1145–53.

10. Mavissakalian M, Brady S. The current state of biologic therapies for treatment of refractory asthma. Clin Rev Allergy Immunol 2020.

11. Loureiro CC, Amaral L, Ferreira JA, et al. Omalizumab for severe asthma: beyond allergic asthma. Biomed Res Int 2018;2018:3254094.

12. Ledford D, Busse W, Trzaskoma B, et al. A randomized multicenter study evaluating Xolair persistence of response after long-term therapy. J Allergy Clin Immunol 2017;140(1):162–9.e2.

13. Tabatabaian F, Ledford DK. Omalizumab for severe asthma: toward personalized treatment based on biomarker profile and clinical history. J Asthma Allergy 2018; 11:53–61.

14. MacGlashan DW, Bochner BS, Adelman DC, et al. Down-regulation of Fc(epsilon) RI expression on human basophils during in vivo treatment of atopic patients with anti-IgE antibody. J Immunol 1997;158(3):1438–45.

15. Chan MA, Gigliotti NM, Dotson AL, et al. Omalizumab may decrease IgE synthesis by targeting membrane IgE+ human B cells. Clin Transl Allergy 2013; 3(1):1–8.

16. Al Said A, Cushen B, Costello RW. Targeting patients with asthma for omalizumab therapy: choosing the right patient to get the best value for money. Ther Adv Chronic Dis 2017;8:31–45. SAGE Publications Ltd.

17. Hanania NA, Wenzel S, Rosen K, et al. Exploring the effects of omalizumab in allergic asthma: an analysis of biomarkers in the EXTRA study. Am J Respir Crit Care Med 2013;187:804–11.

18. Humbert M, Taillé C, Mala L. Omalizumab effectiveness in patients with severe allergic asthma according to blood eosinophil count: the STELLAIR study. Eur Respir J 2018;51 [pii:1702523].

19. Caminati M, Vianello A, Chieco Bianchi F, et al, NEONET Study Group. Relevance of Th2 markers in the assessment and therapeutic management of severe allergic asthma: a real life perspective. J Investig Allergol Clin Immunol 2020;30(1):35–41.

20. Caminati M, Senna G, Guerriero M, et al. Omalizumab for severe allergic asthma in clinical trials and real-life studies: what we know and what we should address. Pulm Pharmacol Ther 2015;31:28–35.

21. Rodrigo GJ, Neffen H, Castro-Rodriguez JA. Efficacy and safety of subcutaneous omalizumab vs placebo as add-on therapy to corticosteroids for children and adults with asthma: a systematic review. Chest 2011;139(1):28–35.

22. Garcia G, Magnan A, Chiron R, et al. A proof-of-concept, randomized, controlled trial of omalizumab in patients with severe, difficult-to-control, nonatopic asthma. Chest 2013;144(2):411–9.

23. Pelaia C, Vatrella A, Busceti MT, et al. Severe eosinophilic asthma: from the pathogenic role of interleukin-5 to the therapeutic action of mepolizumab. Drug Des Devel Ther 2017;11:3137–44.

24. Menzies-Gow A, Flood-Page P, Sehmi R, et al. Anti-IL-5 (mepolizu- mab) therapy induces bone marrow eosinophil maturational arrest and decreases eosinophil progenitors in the bronchial mucosa of atopic asthmatics. J Allergy Clin Immunol 2003;111(4):714–9.

25. Flood-Page PT, Menzies-Gow AN, Kay AB, et al. Eosinophil's role remains uncertain as anti-interleukin-5 only partially depletes numbers in asth- matic airway. Am J Respir Crit Care Med 2003;167(2):199–204.

26. Haldar P, Brightling CE, Singapuri A, et al. Outcomes after cessation of mepolizumab therapy in severe eosinophilic asthma: a 12-month follow-up analysis. J Allergy Clin Immunol 2014;133(3):921–3.

27. Pavord ID, Korn S, Howarth P, et al. Mepolizumab for severe eosinophilic asthma (DREAM): a multicentre, double-blind, placebo-controlled trial. Lancet 2012; 380(9842):651–9.

28. Ortega HG, Yancey SW, Mayer B, et al. Severe eosinophilic asthma treated with mepolizumab stratified by baseline eosinophil thresh- olds: a secondary analysis of the DREAM and MENSA studies. Lancet Respir Med 2016;4(7):549–56.

29. Caminati M, Cegolon L, Vianello A, et al. Mepolizumab for severe eosinophilic asthma: a real-world snapshot on clinical markers and timing of response. Expert Rev Respir Med 2019;13:1205–12.

30. Chan R, Kuo CR, Lipworth B. Disconnect between effects of mepolizumab on severe eosinophilic asthma and chronic rhinosinusitis with nasal polyps. J Allergy Clin Immunol Pract 2020;8(5):1714–6.

31. Hillas G, Fouka E, Papaioannou AI. Antibodies targeting the interleukin-5 signaling pathway used as add-on therapy for patients with severe eosinophilic asthma: a review of the mechanism of action, efficacy, and safety of the subcutaneously administered agents, mepolizumab and benralizumab. Expert Rev Respir Med 2020;23:1–13.

32. Bel EH, Wenzel SE, Thompson PJ, et al. SIRIUS Investigators. Oral glucocorticoid-sparing effect of mepolizumab in eosinophilic asthma. N Engl J Med 2014;371:1189–97.

33. Ortega HG, Liu MC, Pavord ID, et al. MENSA Investigators. Mepolizumab treatment in patients with severe eosinophilic asthma. N Engl J Med 2014;371: 1198–207.

34. Chupp GL, Bradford ES, Albers FC, et al. Efficacy of mepolizumab add-on therapy on health-related quality of life and markers of asthma control in severe eosinophilic asthma (MUSCA): a randomised, double-blind, placebo-controlled, parallel-group, multicentre, phase 3b trial. Lancet Respir Med 2017;5:390–400.

35. Mukherjee M, Aleman Paramo F, Kjarsgaard M, et al. Weight-adjusted intravenous reslizumab in severe asthma with inadequate response to fixed-dose subcutaneous mepolizumab. Am J Respir Crit Care Med 2018;197:38–46.

36. Prazma CM, Katial R, Howarth P, et al. Rigor is needed when making comparative analyses of biologics in severe asthma. Am J Respir Crit Care Med 2018;197: 1508–10.

37. Castro M, Zangrilli J, Wechsler ME, et al. Reslizumab for inadequately controlled asthma with elevated blood eosinophil counts: results from two multicentre,

parallel, double- blind, randomised, placebo-controlled, phase 3 trials. Lancet Respir Med 2015;3:355–66.

38. Bjermer L, Lemiere C, Maspero J, et al. Reslizumab for inadequately controlled asthma with elevated blood eosinophil levels: a randomized phase 3 study. Chest 2016;150:789–98.

39. Kolbeck R, Kozhich A, Koike M, et al. MEDI-563, a humanized anti- IL-5 receptor α mAb with enhanced antibody-dependent cell- mediated cytotoxicity function. J Allergy Clin Immunol 2010;125:1344–53.

40. Tan L, Godor D, Bratt J, et al. Benralizumab: a unique IL-5 inhibitor for severe asthma. J Asthma Allergy 2016;9:71–81.

41. Caminati M, Bagnasco D, Vaia R, et al. New horizons for the treatment of severe, eosinophilic asthma: benralizumab, a novel precision biologic. Biologics 2019;13: 89–95.

42. Bleecker ER, Wechsler ME, FitzGerald JM, et al. Baseline patient factors impact on the clinical efficacy of benralizumab for severe asthma. Eur Respir J 2018;52 [pii:1800936].

43. FitzGerald JM, Bleecker ER, Menzies-Gow A, et al. Predictors of enhanced response with benralizumab for patients with severe asthma: pooled analysis of the SIROCCO and CALIMA studies. Lancet Respir Med 2018;6:51–64.

44. Bleecker ER, FitzGerald JM, Chanez P, et al, SIROCCO study investigators. Efficacy and safety of benralizumab for patients with severe asthma uncontrolled with high-dosage inhaled corticosteroids and long-acting β2-agonists (SIROCCO): a randomised, multicentre, placebo-controlled phase 3 trial. Lancet 2016;388(10056):2115–27.

45. FitzGerald JM, Bleecker ER, Nair P, et al. Benralizumab, an anti- interleukin-5 receptor α monoclonal antibody, as add-on treatment for patients with severe, uncontrolled, eosinophilic asthma (CALIMA): a randomised, double-blind, placebo-controlled phase 3 trial. Lancet 2016;388(10056):2128–41.

46. Nair P, Wenzel S, Rabe KF, et al. Oral glucocorticoid–sparing effect of benralizumab in severe asthma. N Engl J Med 2017;376(25):2448–58.

47. Ferguson GT, FitzGerald JM, Bleecker ER, et al. Benralizumab for patients with mild to moderate, persistent asthma (BISE): a rando- mised, double-blind, placebo-controlled, phase 3 trial. Lancet Respir Med 2017;5(7):568–76.

48. Nowak RM, Parker JM, Silverman RA, et al. A randomized trial of benralizumab, an antiinterleukin 5 receptor alpha monoclonal antibody, after acute asthma. Am J Emerg Med 2015;33:14–20.

49. Deeks ED. Dupilumab: a review in moderate to severe asthma. Drugs 2019; 79(17):1885–95.

50. Castro M, Corren J, Pavord ID, et al. Dupilumab efficacy and safety in moderate-to-severe uncontrolled asthma. N Engl J Med 2018;378(26):2486–96.

51. Wenzel S, Castro M, Corren J, et al. Dupilumab efficacy and safety in adults with uncontrolled persistent asthma despite use of medium-to-high-dose inhaled corticosteroids plus a long-acting β2 agonist: a randomised double-blind placebo-controlled pivotal phase 2b dose-ranging trial. Lancet 2016;388(10039):31–44.

52. Rabe KF, Nair P, Brusselle G, et al. Efficacy and safety of dupilumab in glucocorticoid-dependent severe asthma. N Engl J Med 2018;378(26):2475–85.

53. Papi A, Swanson BN, Staudinger H, et al. Dupilumab rapidly and signifcantly improves lung function and decreases infammation by 2 weeks after treatment initiation in patients with uncontrolled persistent asthma [abstract]. Am J Respir Crit Care Med 2017;95:A6444.

54. Castro M, Busse WW, Zhang B, et al. Dupilumab treatment produces rapid and sustained improvements in FEV1 in patients with uncontrolled, moderate-to-severe asthma from the LIBERTY ASTHMA QUEST study [abstract]. Am J Respir Crit Care Med 2018;197:A6163.

55. Caminati M, Pham DL, Bagnasco D, et al. Type 2 immunity in asthma. World Allergy Organ J 2018;11(1):13.

56. Verstraete K, Peelman F, Braun H, et al. Structure and antagonism of the receptor complex mediated by human TSLP in allergy and asthma. Nat Commun 2017;8:14937.

57. Gauvreau GM, O'Byrne PM, Boulet LP, et al. Effects of an anti-TSLP antibody on allergen-induced asthmatic responses. N Engl J Med 2014;370:2102–10.

58. Corren J, Parnes JR, Wang L, et al. Tezepelumab in adults with uncontrolled asthma. N Engl J Med 2017;377:936–46.

59. Moussion C, Ortega N, Girard JP. The IL-1-like cytokine IL-33 is constitutively expressed in the nucleus of endothelial cells and epithelial cells in vivo: a novel 'alarmin'? PLoS One 2008;3:e3331.

60. Barlow JL, Peel S, Fox J, et al. IL-33 is more potent than IL-25 in provoking IL-13-producing nuocytes (type 2 innate lymphoid cells) and airway contraction. J Allergy Clin Immunol 2013;132:933–41.

61. Anti IL-33 Clinical Trial Program. Available at: https://investor.regeneron.com/news-releases/news-release-details/. Accessed February 20, 2020.

62. Harari S. Randomised controlled trials and real-life studies: two answers for one question. Eur Respir Rev 2018;27:180080. European Respiratory Society.

63. Bagnasco D, Caminati M, Passalacqua G. Biologicals for severe asthma: what we can learn from real-life experiences? Curr Opin Allergy Clin Immunol 2020;20(1):64–70.

64. Bagnasco D, Milanese M, Rolla G, et al. The North-Western Italian experience with anti IL-5 therapy amd comparison with regulatory trials. World Allergy Organ J 2018;11(1):34.

65. MacDonald KM, Kavati A, Ortiz B, et al. Short- and long-term real-world effectiveness of omalizumab in severe allergic asthma: systematic review of 42 studies published 2008-2018. Expert Rev Clin Immunol 2019;15(5):553–69.

66. Abraham I, Alhossan A, Lee CS, et al. "Real-life" effectiveness studies of omalizumab in adult patients with severe allergic asthma: Systematic review. Allergy 2016;71(5):593–610.

67. Alhossan A, Lee CS, MacDonald K, et al. "Real-life" effectiveness studies of omalizumab in adult patients with severe allergic asthma: meta-analysis. J Allergy Clin Immunol Pract 2017;5(5):1362–70.e2.

68. Del Carmen Vennera M, Sabadell C, Picado C. Duration of the efficacy of omalizumab after treatment discontinuation in "real life" severe asthma. Thorax 2018;73(8):782–4.

69. Bagnasco D, Caminati M, Menzella F, et al. One year of mepolizumab. Efficacy and safety in real-life in Italy. Pulm Pharmacol Ther 2019;58:101836.

70. Pertzov B, Avraham U, Osnat S, et al. Efficacy and safety of mepolizumab in a real-world cohort of patients with severe eosinophilic asthma. Pulm Pharmacol Ther 2020;61:101899.

71. Lombardi C, Bagnasco D, Caruso C, et al. Analysis of the drop-out rate in patients receiving mepolizumab for severe asthma in real life. Pulm Pharmacol Ther 2019;54:87–9.

72. Chapman KR, Albers FC, Chipps B, et al. The clinical benefit of mepolizumab replacing omalizumab in uncontrolled severe eosinophilic asthma. Allergy Eur J Allergy Clin Immunol 2019;74(9):1716–26.

73. Bagnasco D, Menzella F, Caminati M, et al. Efficacy of mepolizumab in patients with previous omalizumab treatment failure: real-life observation. Allergy 2019; 74(12):2539–41. Blackwell Publishing Ltd.

74. Bruno S, Gianna C, Elena B, et al. Mepolizumab effectiveness on small airway obstruction, corticosteroid sparing and maintenance therapy step-down in real life. Pulm Pharmacol Ther 2020;61:101899. Available at: https://linkinghub. elsevier.com/retrieve/pii/S1094553919302949.

75. Bagnasco D, Massolo A, Bonavia M, et al. The importance of being not significant: blood eosinophils and clinical responses do not correlate in severe asthma patients treated with Mepolizumab in real life. Allergy 2019;75(6):1460–3.

76. Ibrahim H, O'Sullivan R, Casey D, et al. The effectiveness of Reslizumab in severe asthma treatment: A real-world experience. Respir Res 2019;20(1):289.

77. Menzella F, Bertolini F, Biava M, et al. Severe refractory asthma: current treatment options and ongoing research. Drugs Context 2018;7:212561.

78. Narendra D, Blixt J, Hanania NA. Immunological biomarkers in severe asthma. Semin Immunol 2019;46:101332.

79. Ntontsi P, Samitas K, Zervas E, et al. Severe asthma: what is new in the new millennium. Curr Opin Allergy Clin Immunol 2020;20(2):202–7.

Asthma-Chronic Obstructive Pulmonary Disease Overlap

Check for updates

Sunita Sharma, MD[a],*, Sandhya Khurana, MD[b], Alex D. Federman, MD[c],
Juan Wisnivesky, MD[c], Fernando Holguin, MD[a]

KEYWORDS

- Asthma • Chronic obstructive pulmonary disease
- Asthma-chronic obstructive pulmonary disease overlap • Disease severity

KEY POINTS

- Asthma-chronic obstructive pulmonary disease (COPD) overlap (ACO), as the term suggests, is comprised of clinical and biologic features of both asthma and COPD.
- ACO represents a distinct disorder with unique underlying pathophysiology.
- ACO is associated with increased disease severity including increased respiratory symptoms, disease exacerbations, and hospitalizations.

Asthma and chronic obstructive pulmonary disease (COPD) are two of the most common chronic respiratory diseases worldwide. The prevalence of asthma and COPD continues to increase, exceeding 358 million and 174 million cases worldwide, respectively.[1] Asthma is a heterogeneous disease characterized by chronic airway inflammation with reversible airflow obstruction that results in respiratory symptoms that vary in intensity over time.[2] Conversely, COPD is characterized by persistent and progressive airflow limitation that results from an abnormal inflammatory response in the lungs caused by chronic exposure to noxious stimuli like cigarette smoke or biomass fuels (GOLD), 2017 #54}.[3] Asthma-COPD overlap (ACO) is a syndrome comprised of clinical and biologic features of both asthma and COPD.[4] Although increasingly recognized as a clinical syndrome associated with high morbidity, a consensus definition of ACO does not yet exist. Generally, ACO applies to a subgroup of patients with asthma and persistent airflow obstruction (defined as postbronchodilator ratio of forced expiratory volume in 1 second [FEV_1] to forced vital capacity [FVC] of less than 70% of predicted) or patients with COPD that may exhibit variable airflow limitation and/or evidence of type 2 inflammation.[5] Additional investigations are needed to determine

[a] Division of Pulmonary Sciences and Critical Care Medicine, University of Colorado School of Medicine, 12700 East 19th Avenue, MS C272, Aurora, CO 80045-2563, USA; [b] Division of Pulmonary and Critical Care Medicine, University of Rochester School of Medicine and Dentistry, 601 Elmwood Avenue, Rochester, NY 14642, USA; [c] Division of General Internal Medicine, Icahn School of Medicine at Mt. Sinai, 1 Gustave L. Levy Place, Box 1232, New York, NY 10029, USA
* Corresponding author.
E-mail address: sunita.sharma@cuanschutz.edu

Immunol Allergy Clin N Am 40 (2020) 565–573
https://doi.org/10.1016/j.iac.2020.07.002
0889-8561/20/© 2020 Elsevier Inc. All rights reserved.
immunology.theclinics.com

whether ACO represents a distinct disorder with unique underlying pathophysiology, whether ACO patients should be managed differently from those with asthma or COPD, and whether the diagnosis alters long-term outcomes. This article presents data about the clinical features of ACO, current information regarding the underlying pathophysiology of the syndrome, and current understanding of therapeutic options.

DIAGNOSTIC CRITERIA

Patients with persistent airflow obstruction who exhibit features of both asthma and COPD define the subset of individuals with ACO. This subpopulation remains poorly understood, as studies of this condition remain limited. To date, there is no standardized definition of ACO, with varying definitions across studies. Although the term was first used in the 2015 update on asthma management and prevention by the Global Initiative for Asthma (GINA) and the Global Initiative for Chronic Obstructive Lung Disease (GOLD), neither organization provided a uniform definition.[4,6] Instead, the guidelines proposed that patients with equal features of asthma and COPD as defined by the age of onset, symptom patterns, lung function, family history of asthma, time course of the illness, and chest radiograph findings were subjects who had ACO.[4,6] Characteristics of ACO include: persistent airflow limitation (post-bronchodilator FEV_1/FVC of <70%); (b) FEV_1 improvement greater than 12-15% and greater than 200-400 mLs from baseline after bronchodilator therapy; and asthma diagnosis, atopy, exposure to harmful environmental agents, sputum neutrophilia or eosinophilia, and age older than 40 years (**Table 1**).

In 2016, a global expert panel proposed an operational definition for ACO consisting of several criteria. In order to have ACO, patients must have all major and at least 1 minor criteria. The 3 major criteria are: (1) persistent airflow limitation (postbronchodilator FEV_1/FVC <0.70 or the lower limit of normal) in patients at least 40 year old; (2) at least 10 pack/years of tobacco smoking or biomass fuel exposure; (3) documented history of asthma before the age of 40 years or bronchodilator responsiveness in FEV_1 greater

Table 1		
Key criteria for asthma-chronic obstructive pulmonary disease overlap definition		
Major Criteria	**Definition**	**Number of Criteria Needed**
Age	<40 y	3
Persistent airflow limitation	Postbronchodilator FEV_1/FVC <0.7 or lower limit of normal	
Smoking history	≥10 pack/year or equivalent indoor/outdoor air pollution exposure	
Asthma history	Documented history of asthma before 40 y of age or bronchodilator reversibility >400 mLs in FEV_1	
Minor Criteria	**Definition**	**Number of Criteria Needed**
Allergy history	History of atopy or allergic rhinitis	1
Bronchodilator reversibility	FEV_1 ≥ 200 mLs and 12% from baseline on ≥ visits	
Eosinophilia	Peripheral blood eosinophil count ≥300 cells/mL	

Adapted from Sin DD, Miravitlles M, Mannino DM, et al. What is asthma-COPD overlap syndrome? Towards a consensus definition from a round table discussion. Eur Respir J 2016; 48: 664–673.

than 400 mLs. The minor criteria include: (1) a documented history of atopy or allergic rhinitis; (2) bronchodilator response of FEV_1 of at least 200 mLs and 12% from baseline values on two or more visits; or (3) peripheral blood eosinophil count of at least 200 cells/mL.[7] In spite of having this expert panel definition of ACO, most studies to date have used a myriad of alternative diagnostic criteria. Several alternative definitions of ACO from previously published studies include

Diagnosis of COPD with airway hyper-responsiveness or reversibility of airflow obstruction[8]

Diagnosis of COPD with a history of asthma diagnosed before the age 40 years of age[9,10]

COPD with at least one of the following: bronchodilator response of at least 12%, bronchial hyper-responsiveness, or a decrease in FEV_1 of at least 15% after exercise[11]

The variability in ACO definition across studies has resulted in conflicting epidemiologic and mechanistic studies for this subset of patients and highlights a large knowledge gap in the understanding of the pathobiologic mechanisms that underlie this clinical entity. Furthermore, the recent workshop statement from the American Thoracic Society (ATS) and the National Heart, Lung, and Blood Institute (NHLBI) determined that ACO should be considered an airway disease phenotype of mixed features and argued that there is a critical need for additional epidemiologic and mechanistic studies in the patient population.[12]

EPIDEMIOLOGY

Because of the differences in definition of ACO, the reported prevalence of ACO across studies has been variable. Estimates of ACO in the general population are between 2% and 3% worldwide.[13,14] In compiled data from 4 population-based studies conducted in developing countries (Peru, Argentina, Chile, Uruguay, Bangladesh, and Uganda), the population prevalence of ACO was 3.8% overall, varying from 0% in rural Peru to 7.8% in Bangladesh.[15] In studies of patients with airflow obstruction, the prevalence of ACO is much higher, ranging from 15% to 56%.[16] Population-based studies of adults with asthma suggest similar ACO prevalence rates (15% to 55%).[5,11,17] It has also been shown that up to one-fourth of patients previously diagnosed with COPD actually have features more consistent with ACO.[12,18]

RISK FACTORS

Risk factors for the development of ACO in subjects without pre-existing respiratory disease include older age, male sex, and a history of tobacco smoking.[14,19] However, compared with COPD patients, those with ACO are more likely to be female, younger, have less smoking exposure, and have higher rates of several comorbidities such as allergic rhinitis, anxiety, obesity, gastroesophageal reflux disease, and osteoporosis.[14,15,20] Notably, age, pack-years of smoking, lower education, and biomass exposure were risk factors for ACO compared with asthma, nonobstructed, and general population groups, while higher body mass index (BMI) was protective.[15]

NATURAL HISTORY OF ASTHMA-CHRONIC OBSTRUCTIVE PULMONARY DISEASE OVERLAP

Research on the association of ACO with clinical outcomes has produced inconsistent findings, although they tend to show the same or worse outcomes for ACO compared with either asthma or COPD alone. In a large cross-sectional study of 5044 subjects participating in the Latin American Project for the Investigation of Obstructive Lung Disease (PLATINO) study, ACO was associated with decrements in lung function (FEV_1 and FVC) compared with asthma and COPD.[21] Although lung function normally declines every year after early adulthood, in patients with obstructive airway diseases, the rate of decline in lung function over time can be greater than what is expected because of age alone.[22–24] However, the association of ACO with lung function decline has been inconsistent across studies. In a longitudinal study of 6984 young European adults, the rate of decline in FEV_1 over the 9-year follow up study in ACO was similar to that of asthma, but less than with COPD.[25] In a smaller study of patients with obstructive lung disease, Fu and colleagues[16] reported similar rates of decline in FEV_1 for ACO compared with asthma and COPD. Although the impact of ACO on lung function decline is not yet known, the results of previous studies suggest that additional investigation on the impact of ACO on longitudinal lung function is warranted.

Epidemiologic studies demonstrate a more consistent association of ACO with increased disease severity including frequent exacerbations,[26] poor quality of life,[26] and increased use of health care resources[27] including emergency department visits and hospitalizations.[28] One study reported that ACO patients were hospitalized for breathing difficulty at greater frequency than those with other respiratory disorders (6.6% of ACO patients compared with 1.9% of asthma and 0.5% of COPD) in 1 year.[15] In the COPD Genetic Epidemiology (COPDGene) study, subjects with ACO (based on self-reported asthma history in subjects diagnosed with COPD) had a higher exacerbation frequency and had more airway wall thickening on quantitative analysis with computed tomography (CT) scan when compared to patients with COPD.[10] Mortality studies in ACO are also variable, with some demonstrating increased mortality,[29] while others demonstrate decreased [30] mortality; some other studies showed no difference in mortality between ACO and asthma or COPD.[31,32] Because these data demonstrate the significant impact of ACO on morbidity and health care utilization, an understanding of the mechanisms of disease is essential to reducing the health care burden associated with it.

BIOLOGICAL DETERMINANTS AND BIOMARKERS OF ASTHMA-CHRONIC OBSTRUCTIVE PULMONARY DISEASE OVERLAP

The pathophysiologic mechanisms underlying ACO, and indeed the question of its very existence, remain poorly understood. Mechanistic pathways that might otherwise emerge from randomized controlled trials (RCTs) are unavailable for ACO, as most RCTs on asthma or COPD trials exclude patients with overlapping features of these 2 diseases.

Biomarker studies in ACO are limited and have not been replicated in more than 1 population. In the COPD Genetic Epidemiology (COPDGene) study, participants with a history of self-reported asthma were considered to have ACO. In these subjects, immunoglobulin E (IgE) levels were higher in ACO subjects than in those with COPD alone.[10] Furthermore, ACO subjects also had at least 1 positive specific IgE titer compared with COPD controls.[10] Sputum cell counts have also been used as a noninvasive biomarker of airway inflammation and have been extensively studied in the context of asthma and COPD.

In a study sputum cell counts, patients with ACO had increased eosinophil counts compared with COPD patients, but similar levels of sputum eosinophils as those with asthma.[33] Unfortunately, the sputum cell counts did not correlate with the degree of airflow obstruction or bronchial hyperresponsiveness.[33] Thus, the role of sputum cytokines as a biomarker of ACO remains unclear. In another study of sputum inflammatory biomarkers, the level of neutrophil gelatinate-associated lipocalin (NGAL) in sputum differentiated ACO subjects from those with asthma and COPD.[34] Furthermore, sputum NGAL levels correlated independently with the percentage of prebronchodilator FEV₁.[34]

There are 2 potential additional serum biomarkers that have shown promise for differentiating patients with ACO: periostin, a matricellular protein highly expressed in allergic disease,[35] and YKL-40, a glycoprotein secreted by airway epithelial cells.[35,36] In a small study investigating these serum biomarkers in ACO, serum periostin levels were increased in both asthma and ACO, but not COPD, whereas YKL-40 was high in ACO and COPD, but not asthma.[36] Notably, periostin and YKL-40 were significantly increased in ACO compared with asthma and COPD.[36] Finally, metabolites associated with enhanced energy and metabolic burden are dysregulated in ACO patients when compared with both asthma and COPD.[37] Although these biomarkers are of interest in ACO, additional investigations into these biomarkers in well-phenotyped cohorts are needed to identify replicable biomarkers in ACO (Table 2).

Several additional biologic mechanisms have also been proposed to impact ACO susceptibility. In asthmatics, exposure to noxious stimuli, like cigarettes or biomass fuel, can cause fixed airflow obstruction over time[38] due to progressive airway remodeling. Previous studies have demonstrated that cigarette smoke exposure results in increased neutrophilic inflammation in asthmatics who smoke.[39–41] These changes result in airway remodeling leading to fixed airflow obstruction that is characteristic of ACO.[42] Although few data are available to elucidate the biologic mechanisms underlying ACO, several pathways known to be involved in the pathogenesis of asthma and COPD may be implicated in the development of ACO. Mechanistic studies in asthmatic subjects demonstrate a role for interleukin (IL)-6, IL-8, and IL-17A in neutrophil chemotaxis in the airway of smokers with asthma.[40] Also, smoking may result in the proliferation of CD8+ T-cells in the asthmatic airway,[43] which is similar to that demonstrated in the airway of subjects with COPD.[44,45] These mechanisms have been implicated in the development of persistent airflow obstruction[46] and may play a role in the development of ACO.

Air pollution, which is associated with the development of asthma and COPD,[47] could also play a role in ACO, as suggested by a study in asthmatic adults, in which increased exposure to particulate matter PM₂.₅ resulted in an increased risk of the development of this condition.[48] However, additional investigations are needed to determine if these exposures are indeed a risk factor for ACO.

Previous studies have also demonstrated the role of Th2-mediated inflammation in a subset of COPD patients that may also be important in the understanding of ACO. COPD is generally characterized by neutrophil-predominant airway inflammation,[49]

Table 2
Potential blood biomarkers that differentiate asthma-chronic obstructive pulmonary disease overlap

Biomarker	Type	Asthma	ACO	COPD
Periostin[35,36]	Blood	High	High	Low
YKL-40[35,36,55]	Blood	Low	High	High
NGAL[35,36,55]	Blood	Low	High	High
Immunoglobulin E[10]	Blood	High	High	Low

Data from Refs[10,35,36,55].

but a subset of COPD patients have eosinophilic disease,[50] suggesting that this subset may be particularly prone to the development of ACO. These mechanisms are worthy of additional investigation in a well-characterized cohort of ACO patients to identify the biologic underpinnings of this emerging condition.

POSSIBLE THERAPEUTIC OPTIONS

Aside from complicating the effort to determine ACOS pathophysiology, the exclusion of individuals with overlapping features of asthma and COPD from clinical trials[51] has also limited the understanding of how best to treat these patients. In addition to smoking cessation and discussing the importance of vaccinations, evidence-based treatment recommendations for patients with ACO based on existing evidence remain sparse. The recent COPD guidelines suggest that for patients with symptoms of COPD alone, treatment should include long-acting beta-agonist (LABA) therapy. In contrast, inhaled corticosteroids are reserved for those with evidence of asthmatic features.[51] The previously convened consensus panel recommended the use of inhaled corticosteroid (ICS)/LABA treatment for patients with ACO who demonstrate evidence of increased sputum eosinophils.[7] Other recommendations suggest that ACO patients should initially start on ICS therapy with step-up therapy, including LABA and or long-acting muscarinic agents (LAMAs).[24]

The studies of ICS treatment in ACO are conflicting. In an observational study of 125 patients with ACO, treatment with ICS did not decrease exacerbation rates or reduce the decline in lung function caused by ACO.[52] However, in a study of 127 subjects with ACO of varying severity, treatment with inhaled budesonide was shown to improve lung function, decrease sputum eosinophilia, and reduce exhaled nitric oxide (FeNO) in patients of all severity categories.[53] Compared with COPD patients, ACO patients may have an improved response to ICS/LABA combination therapy in improving FEV_1.[54] Thus, they should be considered for treatment with these options. However, well-powered studies are needed to determine the optimum treatment options for subjects with ACO.

SUMMARY

This article highlighted the existing literature regarding ACO epidemiology, risk factors, mechanisms of disease, and treatment options. ACO represents a subgroup of patients with features of both asthma and COPD, who have an increased risk of morbidity and mortality. Additional investigations into the underlying pathophysiology of ACO and inclusion of these patients in RCTs are essential to improve the understanding of ACO and to determine the appropriate therapeutic modalities for these patients.

CLINICS CARE POINTS

- Patients with persistent airflow obstruction who exhibit features of both asthma and COPD define the subset of individuals with ACO.
- Risk factors for the development of ACO in subjects without pre-existing respiratory disease include older age, male sex, and a history of tobacco smoking.
- ACO is associated with increased disease severity including increased respiratory symptoms, disease exacerbations, and hospitalizations.
- Apart from general recommendations of smoking cessation and immunization, evidence to guide specific pharmacotherapy for patients with ACO remains sparse.

DISCLOSURE

The authors have nothing to disclose that is, related to this work.

S. Khurana has research grants from GlaxoSmithKline and Sanofi and royalties from Spinger that are not related to this work. J. Wisnivesky received consulting honorarium from Banook, GSK, and Sanofi and a research grant from Sanofi. S. Sharma, A.D. Federman, and F. Holguin have nothing to disclose.

REFERENCES

1. Disease GBD. Injury I, prevalence C. Global, regional, and national incidence, prevalence, and years lived with disability for 310 diseases and injuries, 1990-2015: a systematic analysis for the Global Burden of Disease Study 2015. Lancet 2016;388:1545–602.

2. (GINA). GINA. Global strategy for asthma management and prevention. 2017. Available at: http://www.ginasthma.org. Accessed February 14, 2020.

3. (GOLD) GIfCOLD. Global strategy for prevention, diagnosis and management of COPD. 2017. Available at: http://goldcopd.org. Accessed February 20, 2020.

4. Global initiative for asthma (GINA). 2015. Available at: www.ginathma.org. Accessed February 21, 2020.

5. Wang YC, Jaakkola MS, Lajunen TK, et al. Asthma-COPD overlap syndrome among subjects with newly diagnosed adult-onset asthma. Allergy 2018;73:1554–7.

6. Global initiative for chronic obstructive lung disease (GOLD). Global strategy for diagnosis, management and prevention of COPD. 2015.

7. Sin DD, Miravitlles M, Mannino DM, et al. What is asthma-COPD overlap syndrome? Towards a consensus definition from a round table discussion. Eur Respir J 2016;48:664–73.

8. Fu JJ, McDonald VM, Gibson PG, et al. Systemic inflammation in older adults with asthma-COPD overlap syndrome. Allergy Asthma Immunol Res 2014;6:316–24.

9. Hardin M, Cho M, McDonald ML, et al. The clinical and genetic features of COPD-asthma overlap syndrome. Eur Respir J 2014;44:341–50.

10. Hersh CP, Zacharia S, Prakash Arivu Chelvan R, et al. Immunoglobulin E as a biomarker for the overlap of atopic asthma and chronic obstructive pulmonary disease. Chronic Obstr Pulm Dis 2020;7:1–12.

11. Kauppi P, Kupiainen H, Lindqvist A, et al. Overlap syndrome of asthma and COPD predicts low quality of life. J Asthma 2011;48:279–85.

12. Woodruff PG, van den Berge M, Boucher RC, et al. American Thoracic Society/National Heart, Lung, and Blood Institute Asthma-Chronic Obstructive Pulmonary Disease Overlap Workshop Report. Am J Respir Crit Care Med 2017;196:375–81.

13. de Marco R, Pesce G, Marcon A, et al. The coexistence of asthma and chronic obstructive pulmonary disease (COPD): prevalence and risk factors in young, middle-aged and elderly people from the general population. PLoS One 2013;8:e62985.

14. Song P, Zha M, Xia W, et al. Asthma-chronic obstructive pulmonary disease overlap in China: prevalence, associated factors and comorbidities in middle-aged and older adults. Curr Med Res Opin 2020;36(4):667–75.

15. Morgan BW, Grigsby MR, Siddharthan T, et al. Epidemiology and risk factors of asthma-chronic obstructive pulmonary disease overlap in low- and middle-income countries. J Allergy Clin Immunol 2019;143:1598–606.

16. Fu JJ, Gibson PG, Simpson JL, et al. Longitudinal changes in clinical outcomes in older patients with asthma, COPD and asthma-COPD overlap syndrome. Respiration 2014;87:63–74.
17. Weatherall M, Travers J, Shirtcliffe PM, et al. Distinct clinical phenotypes of airways disease defined by cluster analysis. Eur Respir J 2009;34:812–8.
18. Alshabanat A, Zafari Z, Albanyan O, et al. Asthma and COPD Overlap Syndrome (ACOS): a systematic review and meta analysis. PLoS One 2015;10:e0136065.
19. Mendy A, Forno E, Niyonsenga T, et al. Prevalence and features of asthma-COPD overlap in the United States 2007-2012. Clin Respir J 2018;12:2369–77.
20. van Boven JF, Roman-Rodriguez M, Palmer JF, et al. Comorbidome, pattern, and impact of asthma-COPD overlap syndrome in real life. Chest 2016;149:1011–20.
21. Menezes AMB, Montes de Oca M, Perez-Padilla R, et al. Increased risk of exacerbation and hospitalization in subjects with an overlap phenotype: COPD-asthma. Chest 2014;145:297–304.
22. Tashkin DP. Variations in FEV(1) decline over time in chronic obstructive pulmonary disease and its implications. Curr Opin Pulm Med 2013;19:116–24.
23. James AL, Palmer LJ, Kicic E, et al. Decline in lung function in the Busselton Health Study: the effects of asthma and cigarette smoking. Am J Respir Crit Care Med 2005;171:109–14.
24. Postma DS, Rabe KF. The asthma-COPD overlap syndrome. N Engl J Med 2015; 373:1241–9.
25. de Marco R, Marcon A, Rossi A, et al. Asthma, COPD and overlap syndrome: a longitudinal study in young European adults. Eur Respir J 2015;46:671–9.
26. Gibson PG, Simpson JL. The overlap syndrome of asthma and COPD: what are its features and how important is it? Thorax 2009;64:728–35.
27. Andersen H, Lampela P, Nevanlinna A, et al. High hospital burden in overlap syndrome of asthma and COPD. Clin Respir J 2013;7:342–6.
28. Kumbhare S, Pleasants R, Ohar JA, et al. Characteristics and prevalence of asthma/chronic obstructive pulmonary disease overlap in the United States. Ann Am Thorac Soc 2016;13:803–10.
29. Diaz-Guzman E, Khosravi M, Mannino DM. Asthma, chronic obstructive pulmonary disease, and mortality in the U.S. population. COPD 2011;8:400–7.
30. Bai JW, Mao B, Yang WL, et al. Asthma-COPD overlap syndrome showed more exacerbations however lower mortality than COPD. QJM 2017;110:431–6.
31. Sorino C, Pedone C, Scichilone N. Fifteen-year mortality of patients with asthma-COPD overlap syndrome. Eur J Intern Med 2016;34:72–7.
32. Wurst KE, Rheault TR, Edwards L, et al. A comparison of COPD patients with and without ACOS in the ECLIPSE study. Eur Respir J 2016;47:1559–62.
33. Gao J, Zhou W, Chen B, et al. Sputum cell count: biomarkers in the differentiation of asthma, COPD and asthma-COPD overlap. Int J Chron Obstruct Pulmon Dis 2017;12:2703–10.
34. Gao J, Iwamoto H, Koskela J, et al. Characterization of sputum biomarkers for asthma-COPD overlap syndrome. Int J Chron Obstruct Pulmon Dis 2016;11: 2457–65.
35. Izuhara K, Barnes PJ. Can we define asthma-COPD overlap (ACO) by biomarkers? J Allergy Clin Immunol Pract 2019;7:146–7.
36. Shirai T, Hirai K, Gon Y, et al. Combined assessment of serum periostin and YKL-40 may identify asthma-COPD Overlap. J Allergy Clin Immunol Pract 2019;7:134–45.e1.
37. Ghosh N, Choudhury P, Subramani E, et al. Metabolomic signatures of asthma-COPD overlap (ACO) are different from asthma and COPD. Metabolomics 2019;15:87.

38. Chung JW, Kong KA, Lee JH, et al. Characteristics and self-rated health of overlap syndrome. Int J Chron Obstruct Pulmon Dis 2014;9:795–804.
39. Boulet LP, Lemiere C, Archambault F, et al. Smoking and asthma: clinical and radiologic features, lung function, and airway inflammation. Chest 2006;129: 661–8.
40. Chalmers GW, MacLeod KJ, Thomson L, et al. Smoking and airway inflammation in patients with mild asthma. Chest 2001;120:1917–22.
41. Siew LQC, Wu SY, Ying S, et al. Cigarette smoking increases bronchial mucosal IL-17A expression in asthmatics, which acts in concert with environmental aeroallergens to engender neutrophilic inflammation. Clin Exp Allergy 2017;47: 740–50.
42. Broekema M, ten Hacken NH, Volbeda F, et al. Airway epithelial changes in smokers but not in ex-smokers with asthma. Am J Respir Crit Care Med 2009; 180:1170–8.
43. Ravensberg AJ, Slats AM, van Wetering S, et al. CD8(+) T cells characterize early smoking-related airway pathology in patients with asthma. Respir Med 2013;107: 959–66.
44. Saetta M, Baraldo S, Corbino L, et al. CD8+ve cells in the lungs of smokers with chronic obstructive pulmonary disease. Am J Respir Crit Care Med 1999;160:711–7.
45. O'Shaughnessy TC, Ansari TW, Barnes NC, et al. Inflammation in bronchial biopsies of subjects with chronic bronchitis: inverse relationship of CD8+ T lymphocytes with FEV1. Am J Respir Crit Care Med 1997;155:852–7.
46. Boulet LP, Turcotte H, Turcot O, et al. Airway inflammation in asthma with incomplete reversibility of airflow obstruction. Respir Med 2003;97:739–44.
47. Desai M, Oppenheimer J, Tashkin DP. Asthma-chronic obstructive pulmonary disease overlap syndrome: what we know and what we need to find out. Ann Allergy Asthma Immunol 2017;118:241–5.
48. To T, Zhu J, Larsen K, et al. Progression from asthma to chronic obstructive pulmonary disease. is air pollution a risk factor? Am J Respir Crit Care Med 2016; 194:429–38.
49. Stanescu D, Sanna A, Veriter C, et al. Airways obstruction, chronic expectoration, and rapid decline of FEV1 in smokers are associated with increased levels of sputum neutrophils. Thorax 1996;51:267–71.
50. Singh D, Kolsum U, Brightling CE, et al. Eosinophilic inflammation in COPD: prevalence and clinical characteristics. Eur Respir J 2014;44:1697–700.
51. Tashkin DP, Peebles RS Jr. Controversies in allergy: is asthma chronic obstructive pulmonary disease overlap a distinct syndrome that changes treatment and patient outcomes? J Allergy Clin Immunol Pract 2019;7:1142–7.
52. Lim HS, Choi SM, Lee J, et al. Responsiveness to inhaled corticosteroid treatment in patients with asthma-chronic obstructive pulmonary disease overlap syndrome. Ann Allergy Asthma Immunol 2014;113:652–7.
53. Feng JX, Lin Y, Lin J, et al. Relationship between fractional exhaled nitric oxide level and efficacy of inhaled corticosteroid in asthma-COPD overlap syndrome patients with different disease severity. J Korean Med Sci 2017;32:439–47.
54. Lee SY, Park HY, Kim EK, et al. Combination therapy of inhaled steroids and long-acting beta2-agonists in asthma-COPD overlap syndrome. Int J Chron Obstruct Pulmon Dis 2016;11:2797–803.
55. Wang J, Lv H, Luo Z, et al. Plasma YKL-40 and NGAL are useful in distinguishing ACO from asthma and COPD. Respir Res 2018;19:47.

Biologics for the Treatment of Food Allergies

Kanwaljit K. Brar, MD[a], Bruce J. Lanser, MD[b], Amanda Schneider, MD[c],
Anna Nowak-Wegrzyn, MD, PhD[a,d],*

KEYWORDS

- Food allergy • Biologic • Omalizumab • Monoclonal antibody • Peanut • Cow's milk

KEY POINTS

- Food allergies are increasing and are a global health problem.
- Omalizumab may be combined with oral immunotherapy for enhanced safety and tolerability of foods.
- Other biologic therapies and small molecule inhibitors may target the type II allergic pathway and play a role in food allergy treatment.

INTRODUCTION

Food allergies affect 2.5% to 8% of children and 5% to 10.8% of adults in the United States.[1–4] One-third of children are allergic to multiple foods.[2] Food allergies may be more severe and undertreated in low-income and minority children.[1,5–7] Food allergy prevalence seems to be increasing, at an estimated rate of 1.2% per decade.[8] This is particularly true for peanut allergy, which had a prevalence of 2% among children in a 2011 US survey, compared with 0.4% of children in a 1997 survey.[2,9] The health care costs associated with food allergies are also increasing, with increased hospitalizations and emergency department visits being reported globally, but not an increase in anaphylaxis-related fatalities.[10–12]

Risk factors for the development of food allergy include the presence of other atopic diseases, particularly atopic dermatitis (AD) or eczema, which can lead to the development of the atopic march through mechanisms of cutaneous sensitization. Allergen introduction through barrier-impaired skin, as is seen in AD, can result in the activation

[a] Allergy and Immunology, Department of Pediatrics, NYU Grossman School of Medicine, 160 East 32nd Street, LM3, New York, NY 10016, USA; [b] Allergy and Immunology, Department of Pediatrics, National Jewish Health, 1400 Jackson Street, Denver, CO 80206, USA; [c] Allergy and Immunology, Department of Pediatrics, NYU Long Island School of Medicine, 120 Mineola Boulevard, Suite 410, Mineola, NY 11501, USA; [d] Department of Pediatrics, Gastroenterology and Nutrition, Collegium Medicum, University of Warmia and Mazury, ul. Oczapowskiego 2, 10-719 Olsztyn, Poland
* Corresponding author. Pediatric Allergy and Immunology, 160 East 32nd Street, LM3, New York, NY 10016.
E-mail address: Anna.nowak-wegrzyn@nyulangone.org

Immunol Allergy Clin N Am 40 (2020) 575–591
https://doi.org/10.1016/j.iac.2020.06.002
0889-8561/20/© 2020 Elsevier Inc. All rights reserved.

of cytokines, such as thymic stromal lymphopoietin (TSLP), interleukin (IL)-33, and IL-25. This can activate type II inflammation, leading to the downstream production of cytokines including IL-4, IL-5, and IL-13, resulting in allergen-specific IgE, and thus sensitization.[13–15] Allergen introduction that begins in the gastrointestinal (GI) epithelium induces regulatory T cells, suppressing allergen-specific responses, resulting in the establishment of mucosal tolerance, which is most often durable and long-lasting.[16] Targeting of these pathways may help in the treatment of food allergies, and if administered early in life, could theoretically prevent development of allergy.

Other factors in the development of food allergy include delayed introduction of food allergens to the infant diet, changes to the modern diet, and antacid exposure, which can all affect the development of mucosal tolerance.[13,14] Delayed mucosal exposure to foods may potentiate risk factors for cutaneous sensitization because of increased environmental food protein exposure, particularly in patients with AD.[13] Other factors that affect the microbiota, such as delivery by caesarean section and early exposure to antibiotics, may also play a role.[13,14] Current strategies for food allergy prevention are focused on early introduction of foods in high-risk infants, such as those with eczema and established egg allergy, with the goal of building mucosal tolerance from an early age before cutaneous sensitization can occur.[15,17] There is growing evidence that early introduction of peanut and possibly also egg and milk can prevent food allergy among the general population.[15,18] However, this strategy is not effective for all children. Some children develop allergy despite successful early introduction with regular consumption, whereas others develop significant sensitization early in life, and are unable to attempt early introduction. In these circumstances, immune dysregulation seems to override the early exposures, and treatments aimed at the targets of immune dysregulation, such as TSLP, which polarizes T-helper (Th) cells to Th2, and the cytokine signaling pathways, such as Janus kinase (JAK) signaling pathways, may alter a type II-skewed immune system. Current biologics available for the treatment of food allergy, such as anti-IgE, are aimed at minimizing clinical reactivity; however, in the future, potential interventions may focus more on prevention of food allergy.

BIOLOGICS IN ATOPIC CONDITIONS

Biologics used in atopic conditions, such as asthma, target immune pathways that are also relevant in the development of food allergy and anaphylaxis. The number of approved biologic therapies for use in allergy and asthma have drastically increased over the last few years, and there are now five approved biologics for use in asthma. The first approved biologic therapy was omalizumab for moderate-to-severe persistent asthma in 2003. Omalizumab is a humanized, monoclonal anti-IgE antibody, and is currently available as a prefilled syringe or reconstituted solution for subcutaneous use. It is a Food and Drug Administration (FDA)-approved treatment of asthma down to 6 years of age, and chronic idiopathic urticaria (CIU) down to 12 years of age. Dosing is individualized according to weight and IgE level when used for asthma, whereas it is fixed at 150 mg or 300 mg every 4 weeks for CIU. Common side effects include headache and injection site reaction. Omalizumab carries a black box warning for a risk of anaphylaxis, including delayed-onset anaphylaxis, and all patients prescribed omalizumab should receive an epinephrine autoinjector. Anti-IgE treatment downregulates expression of Fcε receptors (FcεR) in addition to inhibiting binding of IgE to mast cells and basophils.[19] Basophil FcεRI expression is markedly decreased after 1 week of treatment with omalizumab, whereas mast cell expression of FcεRI is suppressed after 10 weeks.[20] It may also inhibit allergen-specific activation of T cells.[19]

Subsequently, additional drugs have been approved targeting other pathways and molecules in the type II pathway, including mepolizumab, benralizumab, and reslizumab, each of which target IL-5 and its receptor to treat eosinophilic asthma; and dupilumab targeting IL-4 and IL-13 to treat a range of atopic conditions including asthma, AD, and chronic rhinosinusitis with nasal polyps.

BIOLOGICS IN FOOD ALLERGY

There is no currently FDA-approved biologic therapy for use in food allergy. Omalizumab has been studied as monotherapy and as an adjuvant therapy in the treatment of food allergies, in conjunction with oral immunotherapy (OIT). Omalizumab was initially studied in conjunction with OIT for peanut, cow's milk, and hen's egg, but is now also being studied with multiple food allergen OIT. Combining omalizumab with OIT can result in more rapid desensitization, or a reduction in the inflammatory response during up-dosing by increasing the threshold dose of food protein required to elicit a reaction. This increase in threshold is often temporary, and likely does not represent a "cure" for food allergy in most patients undergoing OIT even with the use of a biologic. However, the increased threshold may help eliminate daily anxiety associated with food allergies given a likely decreased risk of reaction from accidental ingestion or cross-contamination. In the future, therapeutics targeting type II inflammatory pathways, and broader signaling pathways may also have a role in the treatment of food allergies, and aid in the development of durable, long-term tolerance.[21,22] Some are currently undergoing clinical trials.

ANTI-IgE MONOTHERAPY FOR FOOD ALLERGY

The first study to investigate food allergy therapy with a biologic medicine was performed in adolescents and adults with peanut allergy by Leung and colleagues,[19] published in 2003. In this randomized, double-blind, placebo-controlled (DBPC) trial, TNX-901, a humanized IgG1 monoclonal antibody against IgE, increased the threshold of sensitivity to peanut on oral food challenge (OFC) when administered every 4 weeks for a 16-week period, without OIT or any other specific immunotherapy. Subjects 12 to 60 years old given the highest dose of TNX-901 (450 mg) had an increase in mean eliciting threshold dose of 2627 mg of peanut protein at exit OFC (approximately equivalent to nine peanut kernels), from a baseline eliciting dose of 178 mg at entry OFC (approximately equivalent to one-half of one peanut kernel). The study drug was never approved; however, results were positive and indicated that monotherapy with an anti-IgE biologic can increase the reaction threshold among peanut-allergic adolescents and adults, although long-term, durable desensitization was not directly studied.

These promising results led to a trial of omalizumab in peanut-allergic individuals by Sampson and colleagues[23] in 2011. The study became a small phase II trial, because it was stopped early from severe anaphylactic reactions during the qualifying OFC phase of the study. Only 14 subjects completed the trial, including a post-treatment OFC. A small subset of patients (n = 4) treated with omalizumab monotherapy demonstrated a threshold of tolerance greater than or equal to 1000 mg of peanut flour compared with placebo (n = 1). Yet, a similar number of subjects experienced reactions with less than or equal to 1000 mg of peanut flour in both groups. Although there was an increase in reaction threshold between the omalizumab and placebo groups, this was not statistically significant. In a larger study of omalizumab, in which basophil allergen threshold sensitivity was used as a biomarker for clinical peanut allergy, treatment with omalizumab for 8 to 24 weeks resulted in absence of or only mild allergic symptoms during open peanut OFC.[24]

In a 6-month, open-label study of omalizumab in peanut-allergic individuals, the mechanism by which omalizumab may be exerting its effect on increased reaction threshold was further elucidated.[25] By performing OFCs early and late in the treatment period, and following associated diagnostic tests, it was determined that basophil histamine release is suppressed early in treatment, whereas mast cell release as determined by skin prick test (SPT) titration is suppressed later during treatment. Clinically, this was seen as a significant increase in threshold dose of peanut-causing allergic reaction (80–6500 mg; $P<.01$) between the early and late OFCs. This suggests that the basophil has a role in acute food allergic reactions and may explain why omalizumab, which interacts with the FcεR on basophils, nonspecifically aids in rapid desensitization to food allergens.[26,27] In one study, this desensitization was sustained 12 weeks after stopping omalizumab when combined with daily peanut consumption.[26]

Based on this body of evidence, including clinical and mechanistic end points, omalizumab was granted breakthrough status by the FDA in 2018 to expedite its future approval as a treatment of severe food allergic reactions. Since being granted breakthrough status in the United States, Fiocchi and colleagues[28] in Italy have published their experience treating patients with severe asthma, while observing its effects on a subset of 15 patients with food allergy. Subjects ranged in age from 8 to 23 years, and either had multiple food allergies (clinical reactivity to at least two different foods) or a single food allergy, but failed OIT. They underwent periodic open OFCs as part of clinical care, including before initiating treatment with omalizumab (unless there was a recent history of anaphylaxis) and after 4 to 6 months of therapy. Of the 23 different foods evaluated collectively, nine patients were able to tolerate full servings of 16 different foods and subsequently consume these foods in their diet *ad libitum* without undergoing induction, and without experiencing any reactions after introduction. They also noted a decrease in accidental reactions experienced while receiving omalizumab therapy by 95.7%. This real-world, observational study has several significant limitations, including a small sample size without sufficient statistical power, and none of these patients discontinued omalizumab because it was being used for long-term asthma management. However, this Italian clinical experience mirrors other published trials and the data are encouraging.[27,29]

OMALIZUMAB AS AN ADJUNCT TO PEANUT ORAL IMMUNOTHERAPY

In addition to omalizumab being studied as monotherapy, which has a nonspecific effect on food allergy, it has also been studied in combination with specific food allergen OIT. The goal of using omalizumab as an adjunct to OIT is to improve the tolerability by reducing side effects of OIT dosing. It can also facilitate more rapid up-dosing and/or the achievement of higher maintenance doses. Most current food OIT studies aim to increase the reaction threshold in subjects with food allergy so they are less likely to experience reactions on accidental exposure.[30] To accomplish this, some OIT protocols begin with an initial escalation day that is similar to an OFC to determine the starting reaction threshold, and then begin OIT dosing with the last tolerated dose or the protocol-defined maximum starting dose.[31] Other studies have used a fixed dosing schedule, including an initial dose escalation day, after which all subjects begin at a low dose (eg, 3 mg of peanut protein) of OIT, which is taken daily at home.[32] All protocols then continue with a build-up period over several months. Up-dosing is performed under observation in clinic, with continued daily home dosing between visits. This is followed by a long-term maintenance phase with continued, regular home-dosing.[30] Side effects observed in a large, DBPC, randomized controlled trial (RCT) phase III peanut OIT study are typical of type I allergic reactions, including oral pruritis, urticaria, and a risk for systemic reactions including anaphylaxis.[32] GI symptoms, including nausea, abdominal pain, and vomiting, are also common, and can occur shortly after dosing or delayed several hours after dosing, suggesting that there may be IgE- and non-IgE-mediated mechanisms leading to GI symptoms.[33] There is also a slight risk for developing eosinophilic esophagitis (EoE) among patients undergoing OIT; however, this has never been systematically studied.[34] Concurrent or pretreatment with omalizumab can improve the safety profile of OIT by reducing the frequency and severity of allergic reactions.[27,29] However, GI symptoms are not significantly improved by the addition of omalizumab, and GI adverse events are the most common reason for subjects to withdraw from OIT studies.[32,35,36]

In a pilot study of six patients with peanut allergy 12 years of age and older, omalizumab was administered for 4 months before initiation of peanut OIT.[37] This resulted in a higher median initial peanut OIT dose, and fewer reactions on dose escalation days, compared with a comparison group that did not receive omalizumab. These promising results led to further studies, including a larger, DBPC trial.[27] Omalizumab was administered before initiation of peanut OIT to facilitate rapid desensitization. This allowed for faster up-dosing, resulting in a larger dose of peanut protein tolerated on the initial escalation day (250 mg) compared with placebo (22.5 mg). These subjects were also able to achieve a higher maintenance dose of OIT, compared with subjects in other studies, which may provide additional immunologic benefits, including the deletion of allergen-specific T cells.[38] Additionally, this higher dose benefit remains even after omalizumab is discontinued, possibly as long as 72 months in a small cohort of seven patients.[27,39]

OMALIZUMAB AS AN ADJUNCT TO MILK AND EGG ORAL IMMUNOTHERAPY

Cow's milk and hen's egg allergies are the most common IgE-mediated food allergies among younger children.[1] Avoidance of milk and egg is difficult because they are ubiquitous in most diets, and they are important sources of nutrition for children, putting these children at risk for nutritional deficiencies and poor growth.[40,41] Given these considerations, although 70% to 80% of children outgrow these allergies,[42,43] there is interest in offering patients a safe and effective method for desensitization to milk and egg.

The most robust study for omalizumab and cow's milk allergy was a DBPC trial including 57 subjects ages 7 to 35 years with confirmed cow's milk allergy.[29] They received omalizumab or placebo injections for 16 months, and milk OIT was started on Month 4 of injections. The study was unblinded at Month 12 when placebo injections were discontinued, whereas omalizumab injections continued for 12 additional months. Subjects were required to reach a minimum dose of 520 mg of milk protein with a goal of 3800 mg. The active treatment group required a shorter escalation period (median, 25.9 vs 30.0 weeks), had a more successful desensitization (88.9% of omalizumab vs 71.4% of placebo group passed OFC), and experienced significantly fewer symptoms during the escalation phase (91.5% omalizumab vs 73.9% of placebo were symptom free). Immunologic changes showed initial increases in the sIgE to milk and casein in the omalizumab group with eventual decreases lower than baseline, consistent with other OIT studies.[44] However, the sIgE levels in the placebo group trended downward from the beginning.[29] There were no statistically significant differences in efficacy, including rates of desensitization and sustained unresponsiveness (after 8 weeks off milk OIT), between groups, despite the improved safety outcomes in the omalizumab group.

An open-label, prospective study in Spain evaluated the efficacy and safety of omalizumab-assisted OIT to milk and egg in 14 children ages 3 to 13 years who had failed conventional OIT.[45] Omalizumab was administered for 9 weeks before OIT was started simultaneously to both cow's milk protein (goal of 6600 mg) and pasteurized liquid raw egg white (goal of 1800 g egg protein, which is equivalent to one-half of an egg). OIT was started with a 2-day rush procedure followed by continued up-dosing over 18 weeks. One week after the goal maintenance dose was achieved, open OFCs were performed, and after 2 months, omalizumab was discontinued. At the OFC while on omalizumab, all patients had achieved complete desensitization. Side effects were all mild, and only experienced in a minority of patients during up-dosing. However, nearly half experienced anaphylaxis with OIT 2 to 4 months after discontinuing omalizumab. A case series from another Spanish group reported three patients who underwent omalizumab-assisted egg OIT, but developed reactions to OIT doses 2 to 4 months after stopping omalizumab.[46] These experiences suggest that longer dosing of omalizumab may be required to maintain the safety benefits observed during up-dosing.

OMALIZUMAB AS AN ADJUNCT TO MULTIFOOD ORAL IMMUNOTHERAPY

Given the growing body of evidence for the efficacy and safety of omalizumab as monotherapy for food allergy, and combined with OIT to some foods, several studies have been undertaken to examine the potential use of omalizumab with OIT to multiple different foods concurrently. An open-label, phase I study demonstrated early success using a rush desensitization protocol.[47] Twenty-five children between the ages of 4 and 15 years were enrolled, and underwent baseline DBPC OFCs before starting omalizumab for 9 weeks, at which point a rush, initial escalation day was performed. Peanut was the most common allergen included in OIT, in addition to milk, egg, tree nuts, grains, and sesame seed. All foods included in OIT were mixed in equal amounts, including two to five foods, starting with 5 mg of total food protein, regardless of the number of foods included, increasing over six doses to a maximum total dose of 1250 mg of food protein. The maximum dose was achieved by 76% of subjects despite 52% experiencing reactions that were all graded as mild. Subjects started OIT dosing with the highest tolerated dose and then returned for up-dosing visits every 2 weeks, up to a maximum of 4000 mg per allergen (cumulative protein dose of 20,000 mg for 5 allergens), which was achieved by all subjects within 9 months. Home doses resulted in reactions in 5.3% of doses, mostly mild, and typically occurring within the first months of dosing, but there was one serious reaction requiring epinephrine. Omalizumab was stopped 8 weeks after the initial escalation day, and no increase in reactions was seen. This study showed that rush desensitization to multiple food allergens could be done safely with omalizumab and has led to two published phase II studies. The first used a similar protocol as the phase I study, including open-label omalizumab for 16 weeks, but investigated the efficacy of two different maintenance doses (300 mg vs 1000 mg of food protein, per food) compared with stopping OIT dosing.[48] Among 70 subjects, ages 5 to 22 years of age, they found a similar safety profile, but 10 subjects were not able to be randomized to one of the three long-term treatment groups, including five who were not able to achieve a maintenance OIT dose of 1000 mg of each food. The combined long-term treatment groups were more effective at maintaining desensitization to multiple foods after stopping omalizumab, compared with a placebo maintenance OIT for

6 weeks. However, 55% of those on the placebo dose could tolerate 2000 mg of at least two different food proteins at the exit OFC, compared with 85% of the combined treatment groups. There was no difference between the two maintenance doses. A phase II, DBPC, RCT has been performed in 48 subjects between the ages of 4 and 15 years comparing omalizumab with placebo for 16 weeks, in conjunction with multifood (2–5 foods) OIT started after 8 weeks of omalizumab.[49] The same end point as the other phase II study was achieved in 83% of the omalizumab group compared with 33% in the placebo group. The placebo group also achieved a lower dose on the initial dose escalation day and took longer to achieve the maintenance OIT dose than the omalizumab group. Safety results were similar to the prior studies.[47,48]

These promising results have led to a large, multicenter, phase III, DBPC RCT of omalizumab and multifood OIT undertaken by the National Institutes of Health/National Institute of Allergy and Infectious Diseases–sponsored Consortium of Food Allergy Research (NCT03881696). This trial is currently underway and seeks to enroll 225 subjects with peanut allergy between the ages of 2 and 55 years, with a food allergy to at least two additional foods (including milk, egg, wheat, walnut, cashew, and hazelnut).

ADDITIONAL BIOLOGIC THERAPIES

In addition to omalizumab, there are numerous other biologic therapies in development, with the potential to treat food-allergic individuals (**Table 1**). Most of these agents are monoclonal antibodies, which have been approved for other atopic conditions and typically target cytokines or other mediators of the type II inflammatory pathway.

Ligelizumab, an anti-IgE monoclonal antibody similar to omalizumab, may provide additional benefits in combination with OIT. Ligelizumab binds to IgE with greater affinity than omalizumab and has been shown to have faster onset and more sustained control of symptoms in patients with CIU. Additionally, unlike omalizumab there have been no reports of anaphylaxis to ligelizumab to date. It has not yet been studied in food allergy, but could be a potential future indication.[50]

In mouse models, a monoclonal antibody directed against FcεRIα (anti-FcεRIα mAb), the high-affinity mast cell/basophil IgE receptor, has been used to achieve rapid desensitization against egg white, although it has not yet been studied in humans.[51,52] In mice, rapid desensitization with anti-FcεRIα mAb was safer and longer-lasting than rapid desensitization with egg white antigen alone.[52] anti-FcεRIa mAb also suppressed anaphylaxis more rapidly than the anti-IgE biologics omalizumab and ligelizumab.[51]

Dupilumab is a fully human monoclonal antibody against the alpha subunit of the IL-4 receptor, which inhibits binding of IL-4 and IL-13. It is FDA-approved for uncontrolled moderate-to-severe eosinophilic or oral steroid–dependent asthma and uncontrolled moderate-to-severe AD in patients ages 12 years and older, and chronic rhinosinusitis with nasal polyposis in adults. It is available in 200-mg or 300-mg prefilled syringes for subcutaneous administration every 2 weeks with a loading dose at onset of treatment when used in AD and asthma. Phase II trials are underway investigating dupilumab for the treatment of EoE.[53] There is a single case report from 2019 of a 30-year-old woman who had resolution of clinical food allergy symptoms while on dupilumab for severe AD. She was diagnosed with corn and pistachio allergy and following six injections of dupilumab, she inadvertently ate pistachios in a salad. She previously experienced an urticarial rash following ingestion of two pistachios

Table 1
Other biologics of interest/therapeutic pipeline

Name	Mechanism of Action	Clinical Trial Phase/Details	Study Results/Immunologic Changes	Side Effects/Comments	PMID
Etokimab (ANB 020)	Anti-IL-33	Phase IIa: 20 adults with peanut allergy and a history of anaphylaxis 6-wk placebo-controlled study Single dose Phase IIb: 300 adults with atopic dermatitis	73% and 57% increases in tolerated threshold allergen dose of active treatment group (Days 15 and 45, respectively) IL-4, IL-5, IL-9, IL-13, and ST2 levels reduced in the active vs placebo arm on peanut-induced T-cell activation Peanut-specific IgE reduced in active vs placebo	Headache in 4 participants OFC did not test for amounts >375 mg of peanut protein Primary end points not met for atopic dermatitis	31723064 31645451
Ibrutinib	Irreversible BTK inhibitor	6 healthy subjects with a history of IgE-mediated allergy to peanut and/or tree nuts 7-d course FDA approved: B-cell malignancies	Effectively reduced mast cell and basophil activation 77% reduction in wheal size of skin prick tests Nonsustained response, participants were back to baseline skin test reactivity within a week of medication discontinuation	In cancer studies, bleeding events in 39% of patients, more severe in 4%, fatal in 0.4% of 2838 patients Fenebrutinib (GDC-0853) is potent, nonselective, covalent BTK inhibitor in trials for refractory chronic spontaneous urticaria	29360526 29484638 29457982
Dupilumab	Anti-IL-4R (inhibits IL-4 and IL-13)	Phase II: peanut allergy Phase II: peanut-allergic patients on AR101 Phase II: EoE FDA approved: atopic dermatitis, chronic rhinosinusitis with nasal polyps, eosinophilic and/or steroid-dependent asthma	Ongoing, no results EoE: dupilumab reduced the peak esophageal intraepithelial eosinophil count by a mean 86.8 eosinophils per high-power field Dupilumab increased esophageal distensibility by 18% vs placebo	Hypersensitivity reactions, injection site erythema, conjunctivitis, and keratitis	31761117 31593702 31505066

Mepolizumab Reslizumab	Anti-IL-5	No trials in food allergy FDA approved: severe eosinophilic asthma	EoE: significant reduction in tissue eosinophilia but limited clinical improvement compared with placebo		25199059
Benralizumab	Anti-IL-5 receptor-α	No trials in food allergy FDA approved: severe eosinophilic asthma Orphan drug: EoE	Blocks IL-5 receptor, inducing target-cell depletion through natural killer cell-mediated antibody-dependent cellular cytotoxicity		31919743 28530840
Tezepelumab (AMG 157/ MEDI-9929)	Anti-TSLP	No trials in food allergy Phase Ia: 113 adults with atopic dermatitis Phase III: 396 adults with severe uncontrolled asthma	≥50% reduction in the EASI at Week 12, although not statistically significant Less asthma exacerbations Decreased blood eosinophil count, total IgE, and FENO		28877011 31549891 30550828
Enokizumab (MEDI-528)	Anti-IL-9	No trials in food allergy Phase IIb: 329 adults with uncontrolled asthma	No improvement in ACQ-6 score, asthma exacerbation rate, FEV_1, or health-related quality of life	Primary end points not met for asthma	24050312
Lebrikizumab	Anti-IL-13	No trials in food allergy Phase IIb: 280 adults with atopic dermatitis Phase III: 2149 adults with uncontrolled asthma	At Week 16, treatment group achieved dose-dependent, significant improvement in EASI scores from baseline Absence of consistent efficacy in asthma trial	Adverse events include URI, nasopharyngitis, headache, injection site pain Lower rates of ocular complications compared with dupilumab Serious adverse events for asthma trial: aplastic anemia and eosinophilia	32101256 27616196
Tralokinumab	Anti-IL-13	No trials in food allergy Phase III: 380 adults with atopic dermatitis Phase III: 2051 adolescents and adults with uncontrolled asthma	At Week 16, treatment group IGA score of clear (0) or almost clear (1) and significant improvement in EASI scores from baseline	Primary end points not met for asthma Serious adverse events for asthma trial: eosinophilia (>1500 cells per μL) and 1 death from urosepsis	29906525 29792288

(continued on next page)

Table 1
(continued)

Name	Mechanism of Action	Clinical Trial Phase/Details	Study Results/Immunologic Changes	Side Effects/Comments	PMID
Ligelizumab (QGE031)	IgG1κ anti-IgE	No trials in food allergy Phase IIb: 382 adults with chronic spontaneous urticaria Phase II: 37 adults with mild allergic asthma	Binds free serum IgE with much higher affinity than omalizumab Higher percentage of patients had complete control of symptoms of chronic spontaneous urticaria in comparison with omalizumab Greater efficacy than omalizumab for inhaled allergen challenges and skin prick test suppression	Similar side effect profile to omalizumab: injection site reactions and erythema No anaphylaxis reported	31577874 25200415 27185571
Toll-like receptor agonists	TLR9 agonist	Murine model	Decrease in gastrointestinal inflammation, reduction in peanut-specific IgE, and increase in IgG2 values Protection from peanut anaphylaxis	No human studies	29968170
Ruxolitinib	JAK inhibitor	Murine model for food allergy FDA approved: intermediate- or high-risk myelofibrosis and polycythemia vera	Decreased the occurrence rates and severity scores of anaphylactic reaction Decreased IL-4 production Inhibited degranulation of mast cells	No human studies for food allergy	24332884

Abbreviations: ACQ-6, Asthma Control Questionnaire-6; BTK, Bruton's tyrosine kinase; EASI, Eczema Area and Severity Index; FENO, fractional exhaled nitric oxide; FEV_1, forced expiratory volume in 1 second; IGA, Investigators Global Assessment; TLR, toll-like receptor; URI, Upper Respiratory infections.

Data from Refs.[50,53,56-58,60-78]

during an observed OFC and had positive SPT to pistachio. A subsequent OFC confirmed her higher level of tolerance while on dupilumab, at nearly 100 pistachios (50 g unshelled). She also underwent an OFC to corn, to which she had a prior history of anaphylaxis and positive testing. While on dupilumab she tolerated 100 g of corn during OFC without any adverse reactions.[54] Dupilumab is currently being studied in peanut allergy. Concurrent phase II studies are comparing the efficacy and safety of dupilumab versus placebo as monotherapy (NCT03793608) and as an adjunct to peanut OIT (NCT03682770).

Mepolizumab, reslizumab, and benralizumab are IL-5-targeted treatments that are FDA-approved for eosinophilic asthma and may have a potential role in treating food allergy. Mepolizumab and reslizumab bind with high affinity and specificity to IL-5, preventing it from binding to its receptor and reducing the production and survival of eosinophils. Benralizumab binds to the IL-5Rα expressed on eosinophils and basophils, hindering access of IL-5 to its receptor and inducing target-cell depletion through natural killer cell–mediated, antibody-dependent cellular cytotoxicity. These anti-IL-5 therapies have been investigated in EoE, and there seems to be improvement in laboratory and histologic parameters.[55] However, symptoms persist in some subjects despite histologic improvement. The anti-IL-5 treatments have not yet been studied in IgE-mediated food allergy.

Newer anti-IL-13 treatments, lebrikizumab and tralokinumab, have been studied in phase II trials of allergic asthma, AD, and EoE. There are currently no trials investigating anti-IL-13 therapies in food allergy.

POTENTIAL FUTURE TARGETS

Additional biologics in development include those targeting IL-33 and TSLP. Both are epithelial cell cytokines, which play a role in T-cell polarization to Th2 cells.

Etokimab, an anti-IL-33 monoclonal antibody, was used in a small, phase IIa, multicenter, randomized, DBPC trial including 20 adults with peanut allergy. Compared with the placebo group, a single dose of etokimab resulted in a significant increase in the threshold dose of peanut protein eliciting a reaction (73% vs 0%).[56] Additionally, etokimab-treated subjects had reduced levels of IL-4, IL-5, IL-9, and IL-13 in CD4+ T cells on peanut stimulation in vitro, and significantly lower peanut sIgE levels compared with baseline. Although the results seem promising, the sample size was small and the maximum dose of peanut protein during entry and exit OFCs was 375 mg (just greater than one peanut kernel).

Another biologic of interest is tezepelumab, an anti-TSLP monoclonal antibody. In a phase II trial, tezepelumab led to a significant decrease in the rate of asthma exacerbations compared with placebo in adults with uncontrolled asthma.[57] It has also been studied in a phase II trial in adults with moderate-to-severe AD; however, it failed to demonstrate statistically significant improvement in measurable eczema area and severity index scores when compared with placebo.[58] Currently, there are no trials investigating tezepelumab in food allergy.

Bruton's tyrosine kinase, small molecule inhibitors, such as ibrutinib and fenebrutinib, have shown the potential to suppress SPT reactivity, although it is unclear if this could also result in suppression of clinical allergy. Bruton's tyrosine kinase is a downstream enzyme that is required for mast cell and basophil signaling. Ibrutinib is FDA-approved for B-cell malignancies. In a study of two patients with chronic lymphocytic leukemia on ibrutinib with a diagnosis of allergic rhinitis and sensitization to cat and/or ragweed, allergen reactivity was reduced while on treatment. One week after initiation of ibrutinib, SPT wheal size was reduced to 0 mm from greater than 5 mm and there was near complete inhibition of basophil activation. However, the response was not sustained, and subjects' SPT reactivity returned to baseline within a week of medication discontinuation. There was no assessment of their clinical allergic symptoms. This same group studied the short-term use of ibrutinib in six adults with peanut and/or tree nut allergy. After 2 days of treatment with ibrutinib, SPT wheal and flare area decreased significantly (76.6% and 86.0%, respectively), but OFCs were not performed. A phase II open label study of Ibrutinib in adults with food allergy is currently recruiting (NCT03149315).

JAK inhibitors have been widely used in rheumatologic, hematologic, and oncologic conditions with FDA approval for rheumatoid arthritis, psoriasis, myelofibrosis, and polycythemia vera. JAK inhibitors target key cytokine signaling pathways, such as IL-4 and IL-13, and their interaction with the IL-4αR. There is emerging evidence of their efficacy from phase II clinical trials in the treatment of AD. Oral upadacitinib and topical ruxolitinib have been studied with significant improvement in eczema area and severity index scores along with itch scores.[59] In food allergy, JAK inhibitors have thus far only been studied in murine models. Ruxolitinib selectively inhibits JAK1 and JAK2, and has been shown to blunt anaphylactic symptoms and decrease Th2 cytokines in mice. Daily dosing of ruxolitinib in ova-allergic mice significantly decreased rates and severity of anaphylaxis. The mechanism was identified as multifactorial through suppression of mast cell activation, inhibition of intestinal mast cell hyperplasia, and antigen-specific immunosuppression. An advantage of the JAK inhibitors is that as small molecules, they can be administered orally with once daily dosing.[60] However, JAK inhibitors have several associated toxicities, including immune suppression, increased risk of cancers, and pulmonary embolism.

There are limited data on the use of toll-like receptor agonists in a murine model of food allergy. This approach targets the antigen presentation to the innate immune system. Toll-like receptor-4 and -9 agonists are currently in preclinical trials for peanut allergy and have been shown to decrease the severity of anaphylaxis, while also increasing interferon-γ and peanut-specific IgG1 (the murine equivalent to human IgG4). This favors a Th1 and regulatory T-cell response, although this raises concern for the development of autoimmunity if unregulated activation occurs.[61]

SUMMARY

Current biologic treatment of food allergies aims at protecting against accidental ingestion and increasing food allergen tolerability. Anti-IgE treatment has been used with good success for management of food allergies, and is especially effective when combined with OIT, but is not yet FDA-approved for food allergy. Use of anti-IgE treatment, such as omalizumab, allows for modification of not just a single allergen, but multiple allergens at once, because they share a common pathway via basophils, acutely, and mast cells, long term in the manifestation of clinical reactions. This is important because nearly one-third of all individuals with food allergy have multiple food allergies. Future treatments, including dupilumab, an anti-IL-4 and IL-13 antibody, show promise in reducing type II signaling, and clinical trials using dupilumab for peanut allergy are ongoing. Other potential future treatments, such as oral JAK inhibitors, may offer broader immune suppression of key signaling pathways in type II skewed individuals with atopy, but may also carry an increased risk for significant side effects.

In the future, biologics targeting key players in the type II immune pathways essential in the development of atopic disorders may play a role in the sustained treatment and prevention of food allergies.

CLINIC CARE POINTS

- Omalizumab improves safety of food oral immunotherapy,
- Omalizumab monotherapy may also be an option for select patients.
- Real-world long-term efficacy and safety of these novel biologic therapies for food allergy remain to be determined.
- Costs of the novel therapies may limit real-world application.

DISCLOSURE

K.K. Brar has received research support from Incyte Pharmaceuticals, and National Institutes of Health/National Institute of Allergy and Infectious Diseases–sponsored Atopic Dermatitis Research Network. B.J. Lanser reports serving as a consultant for Aimmune Therapeutics (peanut oral immunotherapy), Allergenis (food allergy diagnostics), GSK (medical education), Hycor (food allergy diagnostics), and Genentech (food allergy therapeutics). He is a speaker for Aimmune Therapeutics (peanut oral immunotherapy). He has received research support from Aimmune Therapeutics (peanut oral immunotherapy), DBV Technologies (peanut epicutaneous immunotherapy), and Regeneron Pharmaceuticals (food allergy therapy). He is a member of the National Institutes of Health/National Institute of Allergy and Infectious Diseases-sponsored Consortium for Food Allergy Research. A. Nowak-Wegrzyn is a member of the Data Monitoring Committee for the clinical trials of dupilumab for peanut allergy and has served on the advisory board for Genentech regarding omalizumab for food allergy as mono or combined therapy.

REFERENCES

1. Liu AH, Jaramillo R, Sicherer SH, et al. National prevalence and risk factors for food allergy and relationship to asthma: results from the National Health and Nutrition Examination Survey 2005-2006. J Allergy Clin Immunol 2010;126(4): 798–806.e3.

2. Gupta RS, Springston EE, Warrier MR, et al. The prevalence, severity, and distribution of childhood food allergy in the United States. Pediatrics 2011;128(1): e9–17.

3. Gupta RS, Warren CM, Smith BM, et al. The public health impact of parent-reported childhood food allergies in the United States. Pediatrics 2018;142(6): e20181235.

4. Kamdar TA, Peterson S, Lau CH, et al. Prevalence and characteristics of adult-onset food allergy. J Allergy Clin Immunol Pract 2015;3(1):114–5.e1.

5. Mahdavinia M, Fox SR, Smith BM, et al. Racial differences in food allergy phenotype and health care utilization among US children. J Allergy Clin Immunol Pract 2017;5(2):352–7.e1.

6. Huang F, Chawla K, Jarvinen KM, et al. Anaphylaxis in a New York City pediatric emergency department: triggers, treatments, and outcomes. J Allergy Clin Immunol 2012;129(1):162–8.e1-3.

7. Bilaver LA, Kester KM, Smith BM, et al. Socioeconomic disparities in the economic impact of childhood food allergy. Pediatrics 2016;137(5):e20153678.

8. Keet CA, Savage JH, Seopaul S, et al. Temporal trends and racial/ethnic disparity in self-reported pediatric food allergy in the United States. Ann Allergy Asthma Immunol 2014;112(3):222–9.e3.

9. Sicherer SH, Muñoz-Furlong A, Godbold JH, et al. US prevalence of self-reported peanut, tree nut, and sesame allergy: 11-year follow-up. J Allergy Clin Immunol 2010;125(6):1322–6.

10. Ma L, Danoff TM, Borish L. Case fatality and population mortality associated with anaphylaxis in the United States. J Allergy Clin Immunol 2014;133(4):1075–83.

11. Tanno LK, Ganem F, Demoly P, et al. Under notification of anaphylaxis deaths in Brazil due to difficult coding under the ICD-10. Allergy 2012;67(6):783–9.

12. Jerschow E, Lin RY, Scaperotti MM, et al. Fatal anaphylaxis in the United States, 1999-2010: temporal patterns and demographic associations. J Allergy Clin Immunol 2014;134(6):1318–28.e7.

13. Renz H, Allen KJ, Sicherer SH, et al. Food allergy. Nat Rev Dis Primers 2018;4: 17098.

14. Lack G. Epidemiologic risks for food allergy. J Allergy Clin Immunol 2008;121(6): 1331–6.

15. Perkin MR, Logan K, Marrs T, et al. Enquiring About Tolerance (EAT) study: feasibility of an early allergenic food introduction regimen. J Allergy Clin Immunol 2016;137(5):1477–86.e8.

16. Du Toit G, Roberts G, Sayre PH, et al. Randomized trial of peanut consumption in infants at risk for peanut allergy. N Engl J Med 2015;372(9):803–13.

17. Togias A, Cooper SF, Acebal ML, et al. Addendum guidelines for the prevention of peanut allergy in the United States: Report of the National Institute of Allergy and Infectious Diseases-sponsored expert panel. J Allergy Clin Immunol 2017; 139(1):29–44.

18. Simons E, Balshaw R, Lefebvre DL, et al. Timing of introduction, sensitization, and allergy to highly allergenic foods at age 3 years in a general-population Canadian cohort. J Allergy Clin Immunol Pract 2020;8(1):166–75.e10.

19. Leung DY, Sampson HA, Yunginger JW, et al. Effect of anti-IgE therapy in patients with peanut allergy. N Engl J Med 2003;348(11):986–93.

20. Beck LA, Marcotte GV, MacGlashan D, et al. Omalizumab-induced reductions in mast cell Fc epsilon RI expression and function. J Allergy Clin Immunol 2004; 114(3):527–30.

21. Scurlock AM, Jones SM. Advances in the approach to the patient with food allergy. J Allergy Clin Immunol 2018;141(6):2002–14.

22. Burks AW, Sampson HA, Plaut M, et al. Treatment for food allergy. J Allergy Clin Immunol 2018;141(1):1–9.

23. Sampson HA, Leung DY, Burks AW, et al. A phase II, randomized, double blind, parallel group, placebo controlled oral food challenge trial of Xolair (omalizumab) in peanut allergy. J Allergy Clin Immunol 2011;127(5):1309–10.e1.

24. Brandstrom J, Vetander M, Lilja G, et al. Individually dosed omalizumab: an effective treatment for severe peanut allergy. Clin Exp Allergy 2017;47(4):540–50.

25. Savage JH, Courneya JP, Sterba PM, et al. Kinetics of mast cell, basophil, and oral food challenge responses in omalizumab-treated adults with peanut allergy. J Allergy Clin Immunol 2012;130(5):1123–9.e2.

26. Schneider LC, Rachid R, LeBovidge J, et al. A pilot study of omalizumab to facilitate rapid oral desensitization in high-risk peanut-allergic patients. J Allergy Clin Immunol 2013;132(6):1368–74.

27. MacGinnitie AJ, Rachid R, Gragg H, et al. Omalizumab facilitates rapid oral desensitization for peanut allergy. J Allergy Clin Immunol 2017;139(3):873–81.e8.

28. Fiocchi A, Artesani MC, Riccardi C, et al. Impact of omalizumab on food allergy in patients treated for asthma: a real-life study. J Allergy Clin Immunol Pract 2019; 7(6):1901–9.e5.

29. Wood RA, Kim JS, Lindblad R, et al. A randomized, double-blind, placebo-controlled study of omalizumab combined with oral immunotherapy for the treatment of cow's milk allergy. J Allergy Clin Immunol 2016;137(4):1103–10.e1.
30. Wood RA. Food allergen immunotherapy: current status and prospects for the future. J Allergy Clin Immunol 2016;137(4):973–82.
31. Hofmann AM, Scurlock AM, Jones SM, et al. Safety of a peanut oral immunotherapy protocol in children with peanut allergy. J Allergy Clin Immunol 2009; 124(2):286–91, 291.e1-6.
32. PALISADE Group of Clinical Investigators, Vickery BP, Vereda A, Casale TS, et al. AR101 oral immunotherapy for peanut allergy. N Engl J Med 2018;379(21): 1991–2001.
33. Goldberg MR, Elizur A, Nachshon L, et al. Oral immunotherapy-induced gastro-intestinal symptoms and peripheral blood eosinophil responses. J Allergy Clin Immunol 2017;139(4):1388–90.e4.
34. Burk CM, Dellon ES, Steele PH, et al. Eosinophilic esophagitis during peanut oral immunotherapy with omalizumab. J Allergy Clin Immunol Pract 2017;5(2): 498–501.
35. Virkud YV, Burks AW, Steele PH, et al. Novel baseline predictors of adverse events during oral immunotherapy in children with peanut allergy. J Allergy Clin Immunol 2017;139(3):882–888 e885.
36. Le U, Virkud Y, Vickery BP, et al. Omalizumab pretreatment does not protect against peanut oral immunotherapy-related adverse gastrointestinal events. J Allergy Clin Immunol 2014;133(2S):AB104.
37. Henson M, Edie A, Steele P, et al. Peanut oral immunotherapy and omalizumab treatment for peanut allergy. J Allergy Clin Immunol 2012;129(2S):AB28.
38. Bedoret D, Singh AK, Shaw V, et al. Changes in antigen-specific T-cell number and function during oral desensitization in cow's milk allergy enabled with omalizumab. Mucosal Immunol 2012;5(3):267–76.
39. Yee CSK, Albuhairi S, Noh E, et al. Long-term outcome of peanut oral immunotherapy facilitated initially by omalizumab. J Allergy Clin Immunol Pract 2019; 7(2):451–61.e7.
40. Christie L, Hine RJ, Parker JG, et al. Food allergies in children affect nutrient intake and growth. J Am Diet Assoc 2002;102(11):1648–51.
41. Liu T, Howard RM, Mancini AJ, et al. Kwashiorkor in the United States: fad diets, perceived and true milk allergy, and nutritional ignorance. Arch Dermatol 2001; 137(5):630–6.
42. Savage JH, Matsui EC, Skripak JM, et al. The natural history of egg allergy. J Allergy Clin Immunol 2007;120(6):1413–7.
43. Skripak JM, Matsui EC, Mudd K, et al. The natural history of IgE-mediated cow's milk allergy. J Allergy Clin Immunol 2007;120(5):1172–7.
44. Rachid R, Umetsu DT. Immunological mechanisms for desensitization and tolerance in food allergy. Semin Immunopathol 2012;34(5):689–702.
45. Martorell-Calatayud C, Michavila-Gomez A, Martorell-Aragones A, et al. Anti-IgE-assisted desensitization to egg and cow's milk in patients refractory to conventional oral immunotherapy. Pediatr Allergy Immunol 2016;27(5):544–6.
46. Lafuente I, Mazon A, Nieto M, et al. Possible recurrence of symptoms after discontinuation of omalizumab in anti-IgE-assisted desensitization to egg. Pediatr Allergy Immunol 2014;25(7):717–9.
47. Begin P, Dominguez T, Wilson SP, et al. Phase 1 results of safety and tolerability in a rush oral immunotherapy protocol to multiple foods using omalizumab. Allergy Asthma Clin Immunol 2014;10(1):7.

48. Andorf S, Purington N, Kumar D, et al. A phase 2 randomized controlled multisite study using omalizumab-facilitated rapid desensitization to test continued vs discontinued dosing in multifood allergic individuals. EClinicalMedicine 2019;7: 27–38.

49. Andorf S, Purington N, Block WM, et al. Anti-IgE treatment with oral immunotherapy in multifood allergic participants: a double-blind, randomised, controlled trial. Lancet Gastroenterol Hepatol 2018;3(2):85–94.

50. Maurer M, Gimenez-Arnau AM, Sussman G, et al. Ligelizumab for chronic spontaneous urticaria. N Engl J Med 2019;381(14):1321–32.

51. Khodoun MV, Morris SC, Angerman E, et al. Rapid desensitization of humanized mice with anti-human Fc epsilon RI alpha monoclonal antibodies. J Allergy Clin Immunol 2019;145(3):907–21.e3.

52. Khodoun MV, Kucuk ZY, Strait RT, et al. Rapid polyclonal desensitization with antibodies to IgE and Fc epsilon RI alpha. J Allergy Clin Immunol 2013;131(6): 1555–64.

53. Hirano I, Dellon ES, Hamilton JD, et al. Efficacy of dupilumab in a phase 2 randomized trial of adults with active eosinophilic esophagitis. Gastroenterology 2020;158(1):111–22.e10.

54. Rial MJ, Barroso B, Sastre J. Dupilumab for treatment of food allergy. J Allergy Clin Immunol Pract 2019;7(2):673–4.

55. Stein ML, Collins MH, Villanueva JM, et al. Anti-IL-5 (mepolizumab) therapy for eosinophilic esophagitis. J Allergy Clin Immunol 2006;118(6):1312–9.

56. Chinthrajah S, Cao S, Liu C, et al. Phase 2a randomized, placebo-controlled study of anti-IL-33 in peanut allergy. JCI Insight 2019;4(22):e131347.

57. Corren J, Parnes JR, Wang L, et al. Tezepelumab in adults with uncontrolled asthma. N Engl J Med 2017;377(10):936–46.

58. Simpson EL, Parnes JR, She D, et al. Tezepelumab, an anti-thymic stromal lymphopoietin monoclonal antibody, in the treatment of moderate to severe atopic dermatitis: a randomized phase 2a clinical trial. J Am Acad Dermatol 2019; 80(4):1013–21.

59. Guttman-Yassky E, Thaci D, Pangan AL, et al. Upadacitinib in adults with moderate to severe atopic dermatitis: 16-week results from a randomized, placebo-controlled trial. J Allergy Clin Immunol 2020;145(3):877–84.

60. Yamaki K, Yoshino S. Remission of food allergy by the Janus kinase inhibitor ruxolitinib in mice. Int Immunopharmacol 2014;18(2):217–24.

61. Virkud YV, Wang J, Shreffler WG. Enhancing the safety and efficacy of food allergy immunotherapy: a review of adjunctive therapies. Clin Rev Allergy Immunol 2018;55(2):172–89.

62. Chen YL, Gutowska-Owsiak D, Hardman CS, et al. Proof-of-concept clinical trial of etokimab shows a key role for IL-33 in atopic dermatitis pathogenesis. Sci Transl Med 2019;11(515):eaax2945.

63. Dispenza MC, Pongracic JA, Singh AM, et al. Short-term ibrutinib therapy suppresses skin test responses and eliminates IgE-mediated basophil activation in adults with peanut or tree nut allergy [published correction appears in J Allergy Clin Immunol. 2018 Oct;142(4):1374]. J Allergy Clin Immunol 2018;141(5): 1914–6.e7.

64. Herman AE, Chinn LW, Kotwal SG, et al. Safety, pharmacokinetics, and pharmacodynamics in healthy volunteers treated with GDC-0853, a selective reversible Bruton's tyrosine kinase inhibitor. Clin Pharmacol Ther 2018;103(6):1020–8.

65. Crawford JJ, Johnson AR, Misner DL, et al. Discovery of GDC-0853: a potent, selective, and noncovalent Bruton's tyrosine kinase inhibitor in early clinical development. J Med Chem 2018;61(6):2227–45.
66. Albuhairi S, Rachid R. Novel therapies for treatment of food allergy. Immunol Allergy Clin North Am 2020;40(1):175–86.
67. Harb H, Chatila TA. Mechanisms of dupilumab. Clin Exp Allergy 2020;50(1):5–14.
68. Ortega HG, Liu MC, Pavord ID, et al. Mepolizumab treatment in patients with severe eosinophilic asthma. N Engl J Med 2014;371(13):1198–207 [Erratum appears in N Engl J Med 2015;372(18):1777].
69. Harish A, Schwartz SA. Targeted anti-IL-5 therapies and future therapeutics for hypereosinophilic syndrome and rare eosinophilic conditions. Clin Rev Allergy Immunol 2020. https://doi.org/10.1007/s12016-019-08775-4 [Erratum appears in Clin Rev Allergy Immunol 2020].
70. Nair P, Wenzel S, Rabe KF, et al. Oral glucocorticoid-sparing effect of benralizumab in severe asthma. N Engl J Med 2017;376(25):2448–58.
71. Marone G, Spadaro G, Braile M, et al. Tezepelumab: a novel biological therapy for the treatment of severe uncontrolled asthma. Expert Opin Investig Drugs 2019;28(11):931–40.
72. Oh CK, Leigh R, McLaurin KK, et al. A randomized, controlled trial to evaluate the effect of an anti-interleukin-9 monoclonal antibody in adults with uncontrolled asthma. Respir Res 2013;14(1):93.
73. Guttman-Yassky E, Blauvelt A, Eichenfield LF, et al. Efficacy and safety of lebrikizumab, a high-affinity interleukin 13 inhibitor, in adults with moderate to severe atopic dermatitis: a phase 2b randomized clinical trial. JAMA Dermatol 2020; 156(4):411–20.
74. Hanania NA, Korenblat P, Chapman KR, et al. Efficacy and safety of lebrikizumab in patients with uncontrolled asthma (LAVOLTA I and LAVOLTA II): replicate, phase 3, randomised, double-blind, placebo-controlled trials. Lancet Respir Med 2016;4(10):781–96.
75. Wollenberg A, Howell MD, Guttman-Yassky E, et al. Treatment of atopic dermatitis with tralokinumab, an anti-IL-13 mAb. J Allergy Clin Immunol 2019;143(1): 135–41.
76. Panettieri RA Jr, Sjöbring U, Péterffy A, et al. Tralokinumab for severe, uncontrolled asthma (STRATOS 1 and STRATOS 2): two randomised, double-blind, placebo-controlled, phase 3 clinical trials. Lancet Respir Med 2018;6(7):511–25.
77. Arm JP, Bottoli I, Skerjanec A, et al. Pharmacokinetics, pharmacodynamics and safety of QGE031 (ligelizumab), a novel high-affinity anti-IgE antibody, in atopic subjects. Clin Exp Allergy 2014;44(11):1371–85.
78. Gauvreau GM, Arm JP, Boulet LP, et al. Efficacy and safety of multiple doses of QGE031 (ligelizumab) versus omalizumab and placebo in inhibiting allergen-induced early asthmatic responses. J Allergy Clin Immunol 2016;138(4):1051–9.

Biologics for Atopic Dermatitis

Mark Boguniewicz, MD

KEYWORDS

- Atopic dermatitis • Biologics • Dupilumab • Immune dysregulation • Lebrikizumab
- Nemolizumab • Omalizumab • Tralokinumab

KEY POINTS

- The pathophysiology of atopic dermatitis includes both skin barrier and immune abnormalities, with type 2 immune deviation central to several clinical phenotypes and underlying endotypes.
- Recognition of the persistent nature and systemic aspects of atopic dermatitis provides a rationale for treatment with a biologic.
- Dupilumab, a biologic that targets type 2 immunity by blocking interleukin (IL)-4 and IL-13 binding to IL-4 receptor alpha, has been approved for patients 6 years of age and older with moderate to severe atopic dermatitis.
- Monoclonal antibodies targeting IL-13 and IL-31 receptor A are in phase 3 trials, whereas other targets include IL-33, thymic stromal lymphopoietin, OX40, and IL-22 and may become part of a precision medicine approach to atopic dermatitis.

INTRODUCTION

Atopic dermatitis (AD) is a common chronic inflammatory skin disease that has become a global health problem.[1,2] The Global Burden of Disease Study showed that dermatitis, including AD, was the leading skin disease in terms of global burden of disease measured by disability-adjusted life years.[3] Epidemiologic studies in the United States have shown prevalence of up to 18% in school-aged children[4] and 7% in adults responding in the Atopic Dermatitis in America survey.[5] In this survey, 29% were classified as having moderate disease and 11% as having severe disease. As a chronic, relapsing pruritic disease, AD has a profound impact on the quality of life of patients and families.[6] In a study of adults with moderate to severe AD, 85% reported problems with itch frequency, 41.5% reported itching greater than or equal to 18 h/d, 55% reported AD-related sleep disturbance greater than or equal to 5 d/wk, and 21.8% reported clinically relevant anxiety or depression.[7] Atopic comorbidities of AD, including asthma and allergies, are well recognized, although identifying patients at increased risk for an atopic march remains problematic.[8] Nonatopic comorbidities, including neuropsychiatric and cardiovascular disorders, are also being reported.[9–11]

Division of Allergy-Immunology, Department of Pediatrics, National Jewish Health and University of Colorado School of Medicine, 1400 Jackson Street, J310, Denver, CO 80206, USA
E-mail address: boguniewiczm@njhealth.org

Immunol Allergy Clin N Am 40 (2020) 593–607
https://doi.org/10.1016/j.iac.2020.06.004 immunology.theclinics.com
0889-8561/20/© 2020 Elsevier Inc. All rights reserved.

RATIONALE FOR BIOLOGIC THERAPY IN ATOPIC DERMATITIS

Historically, AD has been thought of as predominantly a disease of children, often outgrown and treated with topical antiinflammatory therapy in a reactive manner. In fact, AD remains a persistent disease or has new onset in a significant number of adults.[12,13] The pathophysiology of AD is complex and characterized by skin barrier abnormalities and immune dysregulation.[14] The systemic nature of AD has become increasingly recognized with inflammatory changes that can be measured in a blood proteomic signature at an early age.[15] Recent studies point to systemic T-cell activation with expansion of circulating T-helper (Th) 2 and Th22 cells.[16] Furthermore, non-lesional AD skin is characterized by broad terminal differentiation defects in addition to immune abnormalities.[17] Although several clinical phenotypes and endotypes have been described, type 2 immunity seems to be central to all of them (**Fig. 1**).[18] Type 2 immune deviation seems to define a distinct AD phenotype and endotype characterized by more severe disease, with *Staphylococcus aureus* colonization, greater allergen sensitization, and barrier dysfunction.[19] The dysbiosis of the skin microbiome in patients with AD has been shown to be related to altered epidermal lipids secondary to type 2 cytokine dysregulation.[20] Recognition of the systemic nature of AD has important translational implications providing a rationale for systemic treatments, especially those targeting type 2 immunity. Of note, advances in the understanding of disease mechanisms have serendipitously coincided with technological advances, ushering in a new era of targeted therapy for AD.[1] This article discusses the use of biologics in patients with AD.

WHICH PATIENTS WITH ATOPIC DERMATITIS WARRANT THERAPY WITH A BIOLOGIC?

Identifying appropriate patients with AD for treatment with systemic therapy, including biologics, has been discussed in several publications.[21–24] A multidisciplinary expert

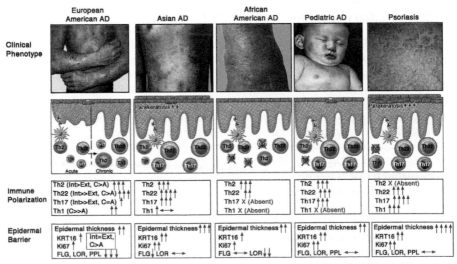

Fig. 1. AD clinical phenotypes and related endotypes. Ext, external; Int, internal. (*From* Czarnowicki T, He H, Krueger JG, et al. Atopic dermatitis endotypes and implications for targeted therapeutics. J Allergy Clin Immunol. 2019;143:1-11; with permission.)

perspective provided a Delphi approach to addressing several key questions, including defining moderate to severe AD as well as treatment failure and recommended a biologic (dupilumab) as a first-line systemic treatment option.[21] The International Eczema Council provided an algorithm for evaluating patients with AD when considering them for systemic therapy,[22] the AD Yardstick added a biologic (dupilumab) to the stepwise management of AD,[23] and a more recent review on managing severe AD included an annotated figure addressing both evaluation and treatment, including with a biologic.[24]

HISTORICAL PERSPECTIVE ON BIOTHERAPEUTICS IN ATOPIC DERMATITIS

Biotherapeutic trials in AD have included treatment with high-dose intravenous immunoglobulin (IVIG), shown to have immunomodulatory effects in AD. IVIG contains high concentrations of staphylococcal toxin–specific antibodies that can inhibit in vitro activation of T cells by staphylococcal toxins.[25] IVIG has also been shown to reduce interleukin (IL)-4 expression in AD.[26] However, treatment of AD with IVIG has yielded conflicting results, with studies that have not been controlled and have involved small numbers of patients and a Grading of Recommendations, Assessment, Development and Evaluation (GRADE) review of systemic therapies found that IVIG was not efficacious in the treatment of moderate to severe AD.[27]

Interferon (IFN)-gamma suppresses immunoglobulin (Ig) E synthesis and inhibits Th2 cell function and treatment of patients with moderate to severe AD with subcutaneous recombinant human IFN-γ (rhIFN-γ), a biologic response modifier that resulted in reduced clinical severity and decreased total circulating eosinophil counts.[28,29] Long-term open-label studies with 50 $\mu g/m^2$ rhIFN-γ given daily or every other day also showed clinical benefit.[30,31] Effective dosing with rhIFN-γ was associated with a decrease in eosinophil counts, suggesting that a subset of patients treated with rhIFN-γ would respond to individualized titration of their treatment dose.[32] Recombinant human IFN-γ has also been used to treat pediatric patients with AD complicated by eczema herpeticum.[33] However, rhIFN-γ-1b is currently not US Food and Drug Administration (FDA) approved for AD.

The observation that patients with AD often have increased circulating eosinophil counts and that products of eosinophil degranulation can be found in their dermis would provide a rationale for targeting IL-5, a cytokine essential for eosinophil growth, differentiation, and migration. However, treatment with mepolizumab, a monoclonal antibody to human IL-5, failed to show efficacy in patients with moderate to severe AD.[34] A limitation of this study was that patients were treated with only 2 doses of mepolizumab over a 2-week period, a regimen that may not have adequately assessed this biologic's effect. Mepolizumab was subsequently studied for a longer treatment period but again did not meet its primary end points despite reducing circulating eosinophil counts.[35]

Rituximab, a chimeric monoclonal anti-CD20 antibody, was shown to be beneficial in a small open trial of patients with severe AD who received 2 doses of 1000 mg by intravenous infusion 2 weeks apart.[36] Histology of skin biopsies showed significant improvement in spongiosis, acanthosis, and dermal cell infiltrates. Expression of IL-5 and IL-13 was also reduced after therapy. Although total serum IgE levels were reduced, allergen-specific IgE levels were not affected. In contrast, treatment with rituximab 500 mg intravenously given twice over a 2-week interval to 2 patients with severe AD resulted in only a transient improvement in clinical scores followed by deterioration.[37] In a novel approach, a small group of patients with severe refractory AD received either rituximab followed by omalizumab or omalizumab followed by rituximab, with positive outcomes suggesting that optimal therapy may require combinations of biologics in select patients, although this would ideally be driven by better understanding the underlying disease mechanisms.[38]

CURRENTLY APPROVED BIOLOGIC

Dupilumab is a fully human monoclonal antibody directed at the IL-4 receptor alpha (IL-4Rα), thus interfering with signaling by both IL-4 and IL-13, 2 key type 2 cytokines (**Fig. 2**).[39] IL-4 binds to type I receptors composed of IL-4Rα-γc heterodimers expressed on hematopoietic cells, whereas both IL-4 and IL-13 can bind to type II receptors composed of IL-4Rα-IL-13Rα1 complexes expressed on both hematopoietic and nonhematopoietic cells. Treatment of patients with AD with dupilumab was shown to suppress molecular markers of cutaneous and systemic type 2 inflammation, as well as reverse epidermal abnormalities that coincided with clinical improvement.[40] In 2 phase 3 trials (LIBERTY AD SOLO 1 and 2), adult patients with moderate to severe AD inadequately controlled on topical treatment were treated with dupilumab, 600-mg loading dose followed by 300 mg weekly or every other week or placebo by subcutaneous injection.[41] The primary outcome of an Investigator's Global Assessment (IGA) of 0 or 1 (clear or almost clear) and a reduction of 2 points or more in that score from baseline at week 16 was achieved by 36% to 38% of patients on dupilumab monotherapy at week 16 versus 8% to 10% on placebo ($P<.001$). In addition, improvement of at least 75% in Eczema Area and Severity Index (EASI-75) from baseline to week 16 was reported in ~50% of patients on dupilumab. Several other clinically relevant outcome measures, including pruritus scores and patient-reported outcome measures, were also significantly improved in the patients treated with the biologic.

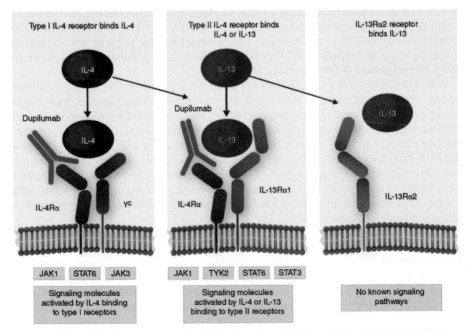

Fig. 2. Type I and type II IL-4 receptors. (*From* Hamilton JD, Ungar B, Guttman-Yassky E. Drug evaluation review: dupilumab in atopic dermatitis. Immunotherapy. 2015;7(10):1043-58; with permission.)

Of note, median disease duration in patients enrolled in the phase 3 trials was ~26 years, median affected body surface area was greater than 50%, and median EASI ~30 (≥21.1 = severe AD). In addition, ~33% of patients had received systemic corticosteroids and ~30% had been treated with systemic immunosuppressives. A critical clinical concept that was not immediately appreciated was that a significant number of patients treated with dupilumab who did not achieve the primary end point of IGA 0 or 1 (clear or almost clear) still had marked improvement as assessed by both investigator-reported and patient-reported validated measures compared with placebo: EASI (−48·9% vs −11·3%, P<.001), pruritus Numerical Rating Scale (NRS) (−35·2% vs −9·1%, P<.001), affected Body Surface Area (BSA) (−23·1% vs −4·5%, P<.001), Patient Oriented Eczema Measure (POEM) score greater than or equal to 4-point improvement (57·4% vs 21·0%, P<.001), and Dermatology Life Quality Index score greater than or equal to 4-point improvement (59·3% vs 24·4%, P<.001).[42] A 52-week study with dupilumab used together with topical steroids (LIBERTY AD CHRONOS) reproduced both the efficacy and safety of the monotherapy trials, showing sustained benefit over an extended period of time.[43] An additional trial in adults with AD with inadequate response to or intolerance of Cyclosporine A (CsA), or for whom CsA treatment was medically inadvisable (LIBERY AD CAFÉ), also provided similar efficacy and safety data.[44]

Injection-site reactions and conjunctivitis were more frequent in the dupilumab-treated patients than in the placebo groups. Although the conjunctivitis has not been fully explained, it was for the most part self-limited, and only 1 patient in the phase 3 monotherapy trials discontinued study treatment.[41] A recent review of randomized placebo-controlled trials of dupilumab in AD (n = 2629), asthma (n = 2876), chronic rhinosinusitis with nasal polyps (CRSwNP) (n = 60), and eosinophilic esophagitis (EoE) (n = 47) found that the incidence of conjunctivitis was greater with dupilumab treatment in most AD trials but very low and similar to that seen in placebo-treated patients in the asthma, CRSwNP, and EoE trials.[45] Greater baseline AD disease severity and history of prior conjunctivitis were associated with increased conjunctivitis incidence. Of note, conjunctivitis was mostly mild to moderate in severity, and most cases recovered or resolved while continuing on dupilumab. Common treatments included ophthalmic corticosteroids, antibiotics, and antihistamines or mast cell stabilizers. Several studies aim to address the underlying pathomechanisms of conjunctivitis in patients with AD treated with dupilumab, including the role of goblet cells (NCT04276623) and cytokine profile of tears (NCT04066998).

As with any new systemic therapy, dupilumab trials were monitored for any signals of increased infections, although the mechanism of action targeting type 2 immunity suggested the potential to correct both immune and epidermal abnormalities.[40] Data from the large phase 3 trials were reassuring, but reflected only 16 weeks of exposure.[41] The 52-week trial provided further reassurance to clinicians,[43] and ongoing long-term open extension studies continue to add to the safety profile of this biologic.[46] In a randomized, double-blinded, placebo-controlled study in adults with AD, dupilumab was shown not to adversely affect antibody responses to vaccines (Tdap and quadrivalent meningococcal polysaccharide).[47] Recently published data from a blinded, placebo-controlled trial showed that patients treated with dupilumab had decreased S aureus colonization and increased microbial diversity that correlated with clinical improvement of AD and biomarkers of type 2 immunity.[48] In addition, in an analysis of pooled data from 7 randomized, placebo-controlled dupilumab trials in 2932 adults with moderate to severe AD, serious infections were reduced with dupilumab, as were bacterial and other nonherpetic skin infections.[49] Although herpesviral infection rates overall were slightly higher with dupilumab than placebo, clinically important herpesviral infections (eczema herpeticum, herpes zoster) were less common with dupilumab. Systemic antiinfective medication use was lower in dupilumab-treated patients.

Subsequently, a randomized, double-blind, parallel-group, phase 3 clinical trial (LIBERTY AD ADOL) was conducted in the United States and Canada in 251 adolescent patients aged 12 to 17 years with moderate to severe AD.[50] In this monotherapy trial, patients were stratified by severity and body weight to 16 weeks of treatment with 1 of 4 regimens: dupilumab 400-mg loading dose, then 200 mg every 2 weeks (baseline weight <60 kg); dupilumab 600-mg loading dose, then 300 mg (baseline weight ≥60 kg) every 2 weeks; dupilumab 600-mg loading dose, then 300 mg every 4 weeks; or placebo with all patients receiving injections every 2 weeks to maintain study blinding. A significantly higher proportion of patients treated with both dupilumab regimens achieved EASI-75 and IGA 0 or 1 at week 16 versus placebo-treated patients. Efficacy of the every-2-weeks regimen was generally superior to the every-4-weeks regimen. The incidence of conjunctivitis in the dupilumab-treated patients (~10%) was similar to that seen in the adult trials. A poshoc subgroup analysis was performed on patients whose IGA was greater than 1 at week 16.[51] Of that subgroup, 80.5% of patients receiving dupilumab every 2 weeks versus 23.5% on placebo experienced clinically meaningful improvements in AD signs, symptoms, or quality of life at week 16. Clinically meaningful improvement in 1 or more of 3 domains of signs, symptoms, and quality of life was defined as an improvement of greater than or equal to 50% in EASI, greater than or equal to 3 points in Peak Pruritus Numerical Rating Scale, or greater than or equal to 6 points in the Children's Dermatology Life Quality Index from baseline. Similar to the adult experience,[42] these data point to the limitations of using IGA as a primary outcome in AD. On May 26, 2020 the FDA approved dupilumab in children 6-11 years with moderate-to-severe atopic dermatitis with weight based dosing by subcutaneous injection: 15 to < 30 kg, 600 mg initial dose, then 300 mg Q4weeks; 30 to <60kg, 400 mg initial dose, then 200 mg Q 2wks; ≥ 60 kg, 600 mg initial dose, then 300 mg Q2 wks.[52] A study of safety, pharmacokinetics, and efficacy of dupilumab in patients greater than or equal to 6 months old to less than 6 years old with severe AD (Liberty AD PRESCHOOL) is currently recruiting (NCT03346434). In addition, pediatric patients with AD have been treated with dupilumab prescribed off label.[53,54]

Dupilumab is approved in the United States for patients aged greater than or equal to 12 years with moderate to severe AD uncontrolled by topical prescription medicines or when those medications are not advised. The approved dosing regimen in adults and in adolescents greater than or equal to 60 kg is a 600-mg loading dose subcutaneously followed by 300 mg subcutaneously every 2 weeks. In adolescents less than 60 kg, the dosing regimen is a 400-mg loading dose subcutaneously followed by 300 mg subcutaneously every 2 weeks. Injections can be self-administered at home, and patients do not require any laboratory monitoring or to be prescribed autoinjectable epinephrine. A study with dupilumab autoinjector has been completed and is under FDA review (NCT03050151). To date, treatment regimens with more or less frequent dosing or stopping and restarting treatment have not been formally studied. One study of patients who had dupilumab discontinued before restarting open-label therapy showed quick recapture of disease control and no adverse events.[46] However, patients could develop clinically relevant antidrug antibodies (ADAs) with repeated stopping and restarting a biologic, and 2 patients with hypersensitivity reactions on dupilumab in the phase 3 trials had high titers of ADA.[41] Of note, patients with AD with comorbidities including asthma and rhinosinusitis seem to respond to treatment with dupilumab as well as those without these concomitant diseases (manuscript submitted). Dupilumab is also being studied in combination with anti–IL-33 (REGN3500) (NCT03736967) as well as with apremilast, a systemic phosphodiesterase 4 inhibitor, as add-on therapy (NCT04306965).

OFF-LABEL USE OF BIOLOGIC FOR ATOPIC DERMATITIS

Omalizumab, a recombinant humanized monoclonal antibody that inhibits binding of IgE to the high-affinity IgE receptor (FcεRI) on the surface of mast cells and basophils, has been used in AD with variable results. Treatment of patients with AD with omalizumab off label has mainly been reported in case reports and case series, showing both clinical improvement and lack of benefit.[55] Specific markers have not been identified that would define responders. Adult patients with AD that responds to treatment have wild-type *FLG* mutations. A systematic review and meta-analysis of omalizumab in AD found that fewer than 50% of the patients treated with this biologic achieved a significant clinical improvement.[56] The 2 randomized controlled trials from that review failed to show significant clinical improvement with omalizumab or the response was comparable with that of the control group. However, the investigators suggested that, because 43% of patients treated with omalizumab had a good response, a subset of patients with AD, possibly those with an urticarial component to their disease, might still benefit from this therapy. Recently, a randomized clinical trial in children with severe AD found that omalizumab significantly reduced disease severity and topical steroid use.[57] As discussed earlier (rituximab), omalizumab may be used in the future as part of a combination or sequential therapy.[38] Of note, a phase 2 trial of ligelizumab (QGE031), a monoclonal antibody with greater affinity for IgE than omalizumab, was completed in 2013 with no results posted, suggesting lack of efficacy in AD (NCT01552629).

BIOLOGICS UNDERGOING EVALUATION IN ATOPIC DERMATITIS

IL-13 is a key type 2 cytokine involved in several pathogenic processes in AD, including skin barrier defects, inflammatory responses, pruritus, and dysbiosis.[58] IL-13 can bind to IL-13Rα1, which, together with IL-4Rα, forms a heterodimeric receptor complex, as well as to IL-13Rα2, thought to function as a decoy receptor that may be involved in endogenous IL-13 regulation (see **Fig. 2**).[59] Monoclonal antibodies targeting IL-13 interfere with IL-13 binding to IL-13Rα1, IL-4Rα, and/or IL-13Rα2. Tralokinumab is a human recombinant IgG4 monoclonal antibody that prevents IL-13 from binding to both IL-13Rα1 and IL-13Rα2. Tralokinumab was studied in a phase 2b, randomized, double-blinded, placebo-controlled, dose-ranging study to evaluate the efficacy and safety of 3 doses of tralokinumab administered by subcutaneous injection in adults with moderate to severe AD every 2 weeks for 12 weeks together with concomitant topical steroids (NCT02347176).[60] At week 12, compared with placebo, tralokinumab 300 mg significantly improved change from baseline in EASI, and a greater percentage of participants achieved an IGA of 0 or 1 and reduction of greater than or equal to 2 grades from baseline (26.7% vs 11.8%). Of note, clinical improvement was greater in patients who had increased biomarkers (Dipeptidyl peptidase-4 (DPP-4) and periostin) associated with increased IL-13 activity. Patients treated with tralokinumab 300 mg showed improvements in SCORAD (Scoring Atopic Dermatitis), Dermatology Life Quality Index, and pruritus numeric rating scale scores versus placebo. Upper respiratory tract infections were the most frequent treatment-emergent adverse events reported as related to study drug in the placebo (3.9%) and pooled tralokinumab (3.9%) groups, with frequency of conjunctivitis 5.9% in tralokinumab

150 mg group and 3.9% in placebo group. This study was confounded by small numbers of patients in each of the 4 treatment regimens and the high placebo response with concomitant topical corticosteroid use. Phase 3 monotherapy trials (ECZTRA 1, NCT03131648, and ECZTRA 2, NCT03160885) for up to 52 weeks in patients 18 years of age or older with moderate to severe AD who are candidates for systemic therapy have been completed, with results pending. In a separate trial, immune responses to Tdap and meningococcal vaccines in patients treated with tralokinumab versus placebo will be assessed (NCT03562377).

Lebrikizumab is another monoclonal antibody targeting IL-13 that selectively prevents formation of the IL-13Rα1/IL-4Rα heterodimer receptor signaling complex. Because its binding is distinct from that of tralokinumab,[61] both monoclonal antibodies targeting IL-13 could be expected to have distinct efficacy and safety profiles. In a double-blind, phase 2 study, adults with moderate to severe AD were randomized 1:1:1:1 to lebrikizumab 125 mg single dose, lebrikizumab 250 mg single dose, lebrikizumab 125 mg every 4 weeks for 12 weeks, or placebo every 4 weeks for 12 weeks after a 2-week topical steroid run-in (NCT02340234).[62] At week 12, significantly more patients achieved the primary end point of EASI-50 with lebrikizumab 125 mg every 4 weeks (82.4%) than placebo every 4 weeks (62.3%), and adverse events were similar between groups and mostly mild or moderate. Again, the study design with mandated topical steroid use limited a proper evaluation of lebrikizumab. Subsequently, lebrikizumab was trialed as a monotherapy using a loading dose protocol in a phase 2b monotherapy trial of patients 18 years of age or older with moderate to severe AD randomized 2:3:3:3 to placebo every 2 weeks or to subcutaneous lebrikizumab 125 mg every 4 weeks after a 250-mg loading dose, 250 mg every 4 weeks after a 500-mg loading dose, or 250 mg every 2 weeks after a 500-mg loading dose at baseline and week 2 (NCT03443024).[63] The primary end point was the percentage change in EASI from baseline to week 16 and, compared with placebo, all of the lebrikizumab groups showed dose-dependent, statistically significant improvement: 125 mg every 4 weeks (−62.3%), 250 mg every 4 weeks (−69.2%), and 250 mg every 2 weeks (−72.1%). Treatment-emergent adverse events were reported in placebo patients (46.2%) and in lebrikizumab groups (48.8%–61.3%), with most reported as mild to moderate that did not require discontinuation. Conjunctivitis was reported in 2.6% of patients treated with lebrikizumab. Lebrikizumab is currently being evaluated in 2 phase 3 trials in patients 12 years of age and older with moderate to severe AD, including a 52-week randomized, double-blind, placebo-controlled, parallel-group study to confirm the safety and efficacy of lebrikizumab as monotherapy for treatment of moderate to severe AD using a 16-week induction treatment period and a 36-week long-term maintenance treatment period using both every-2-weeks and every-4-weeks dosing regimens (NCT04178967) and a 52-week randomized, double-blind, placebo-controlled, parallel-group study to confirm the safety and efficacy of lebrikizumab as monotherapy for treatment of moderate to severe AD using a 16-week induction treatment period and a 36-week long-term maintenance treatment period (NCT04146363). Head-to-head trials of anti–IL-13 biologics versus dupilumab may be needed to answer the question of whether targeting IL-13 alone or both IL-4 and IL-13 is necessary to effectively block type 2 inflammation.[64]

IL-31 is a pruritus-inducing type 2 cytokine that is upregulated in AD, with IL-31 receptor A (IL-31RA) detected in keratinocytes and nerve fibers in the dermis of AD and in the neurons of normal dorsal root ganglia.[65,66] Nemolizumab, a humanized anti–IL-31RA monoclonal antibody, binds to IL-31RA and inhibits IL-31 signaling. In a phase 2, randomized, double-blind, placebo-controlled 12-week trial, adults with moderate to severe AD inadequately controlled by topical treatments were treated with subcutaneous nemolizumab dosed by body weight (0.1 mg, 0.5 mg, or 2.0 mg/kg) or placebo every 4 weeks as well as an exploratory dose of 2.0 mg/kg of nemolizumab every 8 weeks.[67] The primary end point was the percentage improvement from baseline in pruritus visual analog scale (VAS) score at week 12. Treatment with nemolizumab every 4 weeks resulted in changes on the pruritus VAS of −43.7% in the 0.1-mg group, −59.8% in the 0.5-mg group, and −63.1% in the 2.0-mg group versus −20.9% in the placebo group. Improvement in the EASI was −23.0%, −42.3%, and −40.9%, respectively, in the nemolizumab groups versus −26.6% in the placebo group. Changes in BSA involved were −7.5%, −20.0%, and −19.4% with nemolizumab versus −15.7% with placebo. Treatment discontinuation was similar across the 3 dosing regimens of nemolizumab given every 4 weeks and placebo. Although this trial was not designed to definitively compare responses between the dosing regimens, the largest reduction in pruritus at week 12 occurred in the group treated with nemolizumab 0.5 mg/kg every 4 weeks. It is unclear why the higher dose of nemolizumab did not result in incremental benefit. In addition, although the investigators stated that limited size and length of the trial precluded them from making any conclusions regarding adverse events, a review of the data shows that a small percentage of patients treated with nemolizumab developed peripheral edema, pointing to the difficulty in predicting rare adverse events with novel biologic therapies. In a 52-week, double-blind extension study, improvement from baseline in pruritus VAS score was maintained or increased from weeks 12 to 64, with greatest improvement in the 0.5 mg/kg every 4 weeks group with no new safety concerns identified (NCT01986933).[68] Using a different approach, Silverberg and colleagues[69] treated patients with moderate to severe AD and severe pruritus with nemolizumab dosed with either 10, 30, or 90 mg by subcutaneous injections every 4 weeks after a loading dose versus placebo and allowed the use of topical corticosteroids in a 24-week, randomized, double-blind, multicenter study (NCT03100344). When used in combination with topical steroids, nemolizumab improved EASI, Immunoglobulin, and/or NRS-itch scores, with the 30-mg dose being most effective. There was a low incidence of peripheral edema observed in both placebo-treated and nemolizumab-treated patients with no serious cases and 2 subjects treated with nemolizumab discontinued early because of increased creatine kinase levels. A dose-dependent increase in asthma events in patients with preexisting asthma was reported, with mostly mild and very few moderate events that were manageable and reversible. Of note, patients with moderate to severe prurigo nodularis and severe pruritus treated with nemolizumab reported gastrointestinal symptoms, including abdominal pain and diarrhea, as well as musculoskeletal symptoms (NCT03181503).[70] Phase 3 studies currently underway may shed further light on the role of IL-31 in AD as well as rare adverse events (NCT03989349, NCT03985943, NCT03989206). Because targeting of IL-4 and IL-13 also results in decreased pruritus,[41,60,63] head-to-head trials may further elucidate optimal positioning of emerging biologics in AD.

Tezepelumab, a monoclonal antibody, targets thymic stromal lymphopoietin (TSLP), a cytokine that is implicated in the pathogenesis of AD.[14] Epidermal barrier perturbation results in keratinocyte release of several chemokines and cytokines, including TSLP, which in turn acts on group 2 innate lymphoid cells, Th2 cells, and dendritic cells, promoting a type 2 inflammatory milieu, and also directly on cutaneous sensory neurons, contributing to pruritus. Thus, targeting TSLP, which has been called a master switch for allergic inflammation, seems to be strategically important in the present understanding of AD. However, a phase 2a trial of tezepelumab 280 mg or placebo every 2 weeks plus class 3 topical corticosteroids did not achieve statistical significance in EASI-50 at week 12, the primary end point (NCT02525094).[71] Greater-than-expected response rates in placebo-treated patients were likely attributable to topical steroid use. A dose-ranging trial of tezepelumab as monotherapy for AD is currently recruiting and may yield better results (NCT03809663). Although proof-of-concept results from a small study suggested potential benefit of targeting a different alarmin cytokine IL-33,[72] etokimab (ANB020), an anti–IL-33 monoclonal antibody failed to meet its primary end point in a phase 2b trial in AD (NCT03533751). A different biologic targeting IL-33 (REGN3500) is also being investigated as a monotherapy and in combination with dupilumab (as discussed earlier) (NCT03736967). Inhibiting OX40-OX40 ligand interaction could disrupt TSLP-driven type 2 inflammation and a proof-of-concept trial of GBR 830, a humanized anti-OX40 monoclonal antibody, showed improvement in gene signatures and clinical scores.[73] Of note, 2 intravenous doses of the drug administered 4 weeks apart induced significant improvement of tissue and clinical measurements even 42 days after the last dose, suggesting disease-modifying potential.

The Th22 pathway has been shown to be important in AD, with IL-22 participating in epidermal disorder (see **Fig. 1**).[74] By attenuating keratinocyte terminal differentiation and inhibiting tight-junction formation, IL-22 can contribute to barrier dysfunction, and this cytokine's levels are significantly increased in lesional AD skin, correlating with disease severity. A phase 2a clinical trial of fezakinumab, an anti–IL-22 monoclonal antibody, showed significant clinical improvements versus placebo in patients with severe AD (SCORAD>50), but not in patients with moderate AD.[75] A study of fezakinumab that focused on mechanistic responses showed reversal of multiple pathologic features in AD skin biopsies, as well as reduced overall inflammatory burden, not just in the Th22 pathway but also affecting Th1-related, Th2-related, and Th17-related markers.[76] Treatment effects were observed primarily in patients with high baseline IL-22 levels, and, interestingly, participants with low baseline levels of IL-22 had a tendency toward exacerbation of their AD.

SUMMARY

AD is a common inflammatory skin disease that is often persistent and can have recurrence or new onset in adults. Pathophysiology is complex, with both skin barrier and immune abnormalities, including systemic aspects with type 2 immunity central to several clinical phenotypes and endotypes. Dupilumab, a biologic targeting IL-4 and IL-13, seems to correct both cutaneous and systemic abnormalities and has been approved for patients greater than or equal to 6 years with moderate to severe AD. Biologics currently in trials for AD include those targeting IL-13, IL-31RA, TSLP, IL-33, OX40, and IL-22. Further insights into disease mechanisms will help clinicians make more informed therapeutic recommendations as they evolve in the goal to provide precision medicine.

CLINICAL CARE POINTS

- In evaluating whether a patient with AD is a candidate for systemic therapy, define the severity of the patient's AD; review current therapy; and consider alternative diagnoses, as well as concomitant infections, role of stressors, and irritant, allergic, or microbial triggers.
- Before starting a patient on dupilumab, provide education about the chronic, relapsing nature of AD, document severity of the patient's disease, including body surface area involved, and review potential adverse events to be aware of.

- Patients with AD on a biologic may still require treatment with a topical antiinflammatory therapy.

CONFLICT OF INTEREST

M. Boguniewicz has served as a consultant for Regeneron and Sanofi-Genzyme.

REFERENCES

1. Boguniewicz M, Leung DY. Targeted therapy for allergic diseases: at the intersection of cutting-edge science and clinical practice. J Allergy Clin Immunol 2015; 135:354–6.
2. Odhiambo JA, Williams HC, Clayton TO, et al. Global variations in prevalence of eczema symptoms in children from ISAAC Phase Three. J Allergy Clin Immunol 2009;124:1251–8.e3.
3. Karimkhani C, Dellavalle RP, Coffeng LE, et al. Global skin disease morbidity and mortality: An update from the Global Burden of Disease study 2013. JAMA Dermatol 2017;153:406–12.
4. Shaw TE, Currie GP, Koudelka CW, et al. Eczema prevalence in the United States: data from the 2003 National Survey of Children's Health. J Invest Dermatol 2011; 131:67–73.
5. Chiesa Fuxench ZC, Block JK, Boguniewicz M, et al. Atopic Dermatitis in America Study: A cross-sectional study examining the prevalence and disease burden of atopic dermatitis in the US adult population. J Invest Dermatol 2019;139:583–90.
6. Silverberg JI, Gelfand JM, Margolis DJ, et al. Patient burden and quality of life in atopic dermatitis in US adults: A population-based cross-sectional study. Ann Allergy Asthma Immunol 2018;121:340–7.
7. Simpson EL, Bieber T, Eckert L, et al. Patient burden of moderate to severe atopic dermatitis (AD): Insights from a phase 2b clinical trial of dupilumab in adults. J Am Acad Dermatol 2016;74:491–8.
8. Davidson WF, Leung DYM, Beck LA, et al. Report from the National Institute of Allergy and Infectious Diseases workshop on "Atopic dermatitis and the atopic march: Mechanisms and interventions. J Allergy Clin Immunol 2019;143: 894–913.
9. Paller A, Jaworski JC, Simpson EL, et al. Major comorbidities of atopic dermatitis: Beyond allergic disorders. Am J Clin Dermatol 2018;19:821–38.
10. Silverberg JI, Gelfand JM, Margolis DJ, et al. Association of atopic dermatitis with allergic, autoimmune and cardiovascular comorbidities in US adults. Ann Allergy Asthma Immunol 2018;121:604–12.e3.
11. He H, Li R, Choi S, et al. Increased cardiovascular and atherosclerosis markers in blood of older patients with atopic dermatitis. Ann Allergy Asthma Immunol 2020; 124:70–8.
12. Margolis JS, Abuabara K, Bilker W, et al. Persistence of mild to moderate atopic dermatitis. JAMA Dermatol 2014;150:593–600.
13. Bieber T, D'Erme AM, Akdis CA, et al. Clinical phenotypes and endophenotypes of atopic dermatitis: Where are we, and where should we go? J Allergy Clin Immunol 2017;139:S58–64.
14. Boguniewicz M, Leung DY. Atopic dermatitis: a disease of altered skin barrier and immune dysregulation. Immunol Rev 2011;242:233–46.
15. Brunner PM, He H, Pavel AB, et al. The blood proteomic signature of early-onset pediatric atopic dermatitis shows systemic inflammation and is distinct from adult long-standing disease. J Am Acad Dermatol 2019;81:510–9.

16. Czarnowicki T, Gonzalez J, Shemer A, et al. Severe atopic dermatitis is characterized by selective expansion of circulating TH2/TC2 and TH22/TC22, but not TH17/TC17, cells within the skin-homing T-cell population. J Allergy Clin Immunol 2015;136:104–15.e7.

17. Suárez-Fariñas M, Tintle SJ, Shemer A, et al. Nonlesional atopic dermatitis skin is characterized by broad terminal differentiation defects and variable immune abnormalities. J Allergy Clin Immunol 2011;127:954–64.e1-4.

18. Czarnowicki T, He H, Krueger JG, et al. Atopic dermatitis endotypes and implications for targeted therapeutics. J Allergy Clin Immunol 2019;143:1–11.

19. Simpson EL, Villarreal M, Jepson B, et al. Patients with atopic dermatitis colonized with Staphylococcus aureus have a distinct phenotype and endotype. J Invest Dermatol 2018;138:2224–33.

20. Berdyshev E, Goleva E, Bronova I, et al. Lipid abnormalities in atopic skin are driven by type 2 cytokines. JCI Insight 2018;3(4):e98006.

21. Boguniewicz M, Alexis AF, Beck LA, et al. Expert perspectives on management of moderate-to-severe atopic dermatitis: a multidisciplinary consensus addressing current and emerging therapies. J Allergy Clin Immunol Pract 2017;5:1519–31.

22. Simpson EL, Bruin-Weller M, Flohr C, et al. When does atopic dermatitis warrant systemic therapy? recommendations from an expert panel of the international eczema council. J Am Acad Dermatol 2017;77:623–33.

23. Boguniewicz M, Fonacier L, Guttman-Yassky E, et al. Atopic Dermatitis Yardstick: Practical recommendations for an evolving therapeutic landscape. Ann Allergy Asthma Immunol 2018;120:10–22.e2.

24. Brar K, Nicol NH, Boguniewicz M. Strategies for successful management of severe atopic dermatitis. J Allergy Clin Immunol Pract 2019;7:1–16.

25. Takei S, Arora YK, Walker SM. Intravenous immunoglobulin contains specific antibodies inhibitory to activation of T cells by staphylococcal toxin superantigens. J Clin Invest 1993;91:602–7.

26. Jolles S, Hughes J, Rustin M. Intracellular interleukin-4 profiles during high-dose intravenous immunoglobulin treatment of therapy-resistant atopic dermatitis. J Am Acad Dermatol 1999;40:121–3.

27. Roekevisch E, Spuls PI, Kuester D, et al. Efficacy and safety of systemic treatments for moderate-to-severe atopic dermatitis: a systematic review. J Allergy Clin Immunol 2014;133:429–38.

28. Boguniewicz M, Jaffe HS, Izu A, et al. Recombinant gamma interferon in treatment of patients with atopic dermatitis and elevated IgE levels. Am J Med 1990;88:365–70.

29. Hanifin JM, Schneider LC, Leung DY, et al. Recombinant interferon gamma therapy for atopic dermatitis. J Am Acad Dermatol 1993;28:189–97.

30. Schneider LC, Baz Z, Zarcone C, et al. Long-term therapy with recombinant interferon-gamma (rIFN-gamma) for atopic dermatitis. Ann Allergy Asthma Immunol 1998;80:263–8.

31. Stevens SR, Hanifin JM, Hamilton T, et al. Long-term effectiveness and safety of recombinant human interferon gamma therapy for atopic dermatitis despite unchanged serum IgE levels. Arch Dermatol 1998;134:799–804.

32. Boguniewicz M, Leung DY. Atopic dermatitis: a question of balance. Arch Dermatol 1998;134:870–1.

33. Frisch S, Siegfried EC. The clinical spectrum and therapeutic challenge of eczema herpeticum. Pediatr Dermatol 2011;28:46–52.

34. Oldhoff JM, Darsow U, Werfel T, et al. Anti-IL-5 recombinant humanized monoclonal antibody (mepolizumab) for the treatment of atopic dermatitis. Allergy 2005;60:693–6.

35. Kang EG, Narayana PK, Pouliquen IJ, et al. Efficacy and safety of mepolizumab administered subcutaneously for moderate to severe atopic dermatitis. Allergy 2020;75(4):950–3.

36. Simon D, Hösli S, Kostylina G, et al. Anti-CD20 (rituximab) treatment improves atopic eczema. J Allergy Clin Immunol 2008;121:122–8.

37. Sedivá A, Kayserová J, Vernerová E, et al. Anti-CD20 (rituximab) treatment for atopic eczema. J Allergy Clin Immunol 2008;121:1515–6.

38. Sánchez-Ramón S, Eguíluz-Gracia I, Rodríguez-Mazariego ME, et al. Sequential combined therapy with omalizumab and rituximab: a new approach to severe atopic dermatitis. J Investig Allergol Clin Immunol 2013;23:190–6.

39. Hamilton JD, Ungar B, Guttman-Yassky E. Drug evaluation review: dupilumab in atopic dermatitis. Immunotherapy 2015;7:1043–58.

40. Guttman-Yassky E, Bissonnette R, Ungar B, et al. Dupilumab progressively improves systemic and cutaneous abnormalities in patients with atopic dermatitis. J Allergy Clin Immunol 2019;143:155–72.

41. Simpson EL, Bieber T, Guttman-Yassky E, et al. Two phase 3 trials of dupilumab versus placebo in atopic dermatitis. N Engl J Med 2016;375:2335–48.

42. Silverberg JI, Simpson EL, Ardeleanu M, et al. Dupilumab provides important clinical benefits to patient with atopic dermatitis who do not achieve clear or almost clear skin according to the Investigator's Global Assessment: a pooled analysis of data from two phase III trials. Br J Dermatol 2019;181:80–7.

43. Blauvelt A, de Bruin-Weller M, Gooderham M, et al. Long-term management of moderate-to-severe atopic dermatitis with dupilumab and concomitant topical corticosteroids (LIBERTY AD CHRONOS): a 1-year, randomised, double-blinded, placebo-controlled, phase 3 trial. Lancet 2017;389:2287–303.

44. de Bruin-Weller M, Thaçi D, Smith CH, et al. Dupilumab with concomitant topical corticosteroid treatment in adults with atopic dermatitis with an inadequate response or intolerance to ciclosporin A or when this treatment is medically inadvisable: a placebo-controlled, randomized phase III clinical trial (LIBERTY AD CAFÉ). Br J Dermatol 2018;178:1083–101.

45. Akinlade B, Guttman-Yassky E, de Bruin-Weller M, et al. Conjunctivitis in dupilumab clinical trials. Br J Dermatol 2019;181:459–73.

46. Deleuran M, Thaçi D, Beck LA, et al. Dupilumab shows long-term safety and efficacy in patients with moderate to severe atopic dermatitis enrolled in a phase 3 open-label extension study. J Am Acad Dermatol 2020;82:377–88.

47. Blauvelt A, Simpson EL, Tyring SK, et al. Dupilumab does not affect correlates of vaccine-induced immunity: A randomized, placebo-controlled trial in adults with moderate-to-severe atopic dermatitis. J Am Acad Dermatol 2019;80:158–67.e1.

48. Callewaert C, Nakatsuji T, Knight R, et al. IL-4Rα blockade by dupilumab decreases Staphylococcus aureus colonization and increases microbial diversity in atopic dermatitis. J Invest Dermatol 2020;140:191–202.e7.

49. Eichenfield LF, Bieber T, Beck LA, et al. Infections in Dupilumab Clinical Trials in Atopic Dermatitis: A Comprehensive Pooled Analysis. Am J Clin Dermatol 2019;20:443–56.

50. Simpson EL, Paller AS, Siegfried EC, et al. Efficacy and Safety of Dupilumab in Adolescents With Uncontrolled Moderate to Severe Atopic Dermatitis: A Phase 3 Randomized Clinical Trial. JAMA Dermatol 2019;156(1):44–56.

51. Paller AS, Bansal A, Simpson EL, et al. Clinically Meaningful Responses to Dupilumab in Adolescents with Uncontrolled Moderate-to-Severe Atopic Dermatitis: Post-hoc Analyses from a Randomized Clinical Trial. Am J Clin Dermatol 2020; 21:119–31.

52. Paller AS, Siegfried EC, Thaçi D, et al. Efficacy and safety of dupilumab with concomitant topical corticosteroids in children 6 to 11 years old with severe atopic dermatitis: a randomized, double-blinded, placebo-controlled phase 3 trial. J Am Acad Dermatol 2020 [published online ahead of print, Jun 20].

53. Treister AD, Lio PA. Long-term off-label dupilumab in pediatric atopic dermatitis: a case series. Pediatr Dermatol 2019;36:85–8.

54. Siegfried EC, Igelman S, Jaworsk JC, et al. Use of dupilimab in pediatric atopic dermatitis: Access, dosing, and implications for managing severe atopic dermatitis. Pediatr Dermatol 2019;36:172–6.

55. Lacombe Barrios J, Bégin P, Paradis L, et al. Anti-IgE therapy and severe atopic dermatitis: a pediatric perspective. J Am Acad Dermatol 2013;69:832–4.

56. Wang HH, Li YC, Huang YC. Efficacy of omalizumab in patients with atopic dermatitis: A systematic review and meta-analysis. J Allergy Clin Immunol 2016;138:1719–17122.e1.

57. Chan S, Cornelius V, Cro S, et al. Treatment Effect of Omalizumab on Severe Pediatric Atopic Dermatitis: The ADAPT Randomized Clinical Trial. JAMA Pediatr 2019;174(1):29–37.

58. Bieber T. Interleukin-13: targeting an underestimated cytokine in atopic dermatitis. Allergy 2020;75:54–62.

59. Moyle M, Cevikbas F, Harden JL, et al. Understanding the immune landscape in atopic dermatitis: The era of biologics and emerging therapeutic approaches. Exp Dermatol 2019;28:756–68.

60. Wollenberg A, Howell MD, Guttman-Yassky E, et al. Treatment of atopic dermatitis with tralokinumab, an anti-IL-13 mAb. J Allergy Clin Immunol 2019;143:135–41.

61. Popovic B, Breed J, Rees DG, et al. Structural characterisation reveals mechanism of IL-13-neutralising monoclonal antibody tralokinumab as inhibition of binding to IL-13Ra1 and IL-13Ra2. J Mol Biol 2017;429:208–19.

62. Simpson EL, Flohr C, Eichenfield LF, et al. Efficacy and safety of lebrikizumab (an anti-IL-13 monoclonal antibody) in adults with moderate-to-severe atopic dermatitis inadequately controlled by topical corticosteroids: A randomized, placebo-controlled phase II trial (TREBLE). J Am Acad Dermatol 2018;78:863–71.

63. Guttman-Yassky E, Blauvelt A, Eichenfield LF, et al. Efficacy and safety of lebrikizumab, a high-affinity interleukin 13 inhibitor, in adults with moderate to severe atopic dermatitis: A phase 2b randomized clinical trial. JAMA Dermatol 2020; 156(4):411–20.

64. Le Floc'h A, Allinne J, Nagashima K, et al. Dual blockade of IL-4 and IL-13 with dupilumab, an IL-4Rα antibody, is required to broadly inhibit type 2 inflammation. Allergy 2020;75(5):1188–204.

65. Bilsborough J, Leung DY, Maurer M, et al. IL-31 is associated with cutaneous lymphocyte antigen-positive skin homing T cells in patients with atopic dermatitis. J Allergy Clin Immunol 2006;117:418–25.

66. Kato A, Fujii E, Watanabe T, et al. Distribution of IL-31 and its receptor expressing cells in skin of atopic dermatitis. J Dermatol Sci 2014;74:229–35.

67. Ruzicka T, Hanifin JM, Furue M, et al. Anti-interleukin-31 receptor A antibody for atopic dermatitis. N Engl J Med 2017;376:826–35.

68. Kabashima K, Furue M, Hanifin JM, et al. Nemolizumab in patients with moderate-to-severe atopic dermatitis: randomized, phase II, long-term extension study. J Allergy Clin Immunol 2018;142:1121–30.
69. Silverberg JI, Pinter A, Pulka G, et al. Phase 2B randomized study of nemolizumab in adults with moderate-to-severe atopic dermatitis and severe pruritus. J Allergy Clin Immunol 2020;145:173–82.
70. Stander S, Yosipovitch G, Legat FJ, et al. Trial of nemolizumab in moderate-to-severe prurigo nodularis. N Engl J Med 2020;382:706–16.
71. Simpson EL, Parnes JR, She D, et al. Tezepelumab, an anti-thymic stromal lymphopoietin monoclonal antibody, in the treatment of moderate to severe atopic dermatitis: A randomized phase 2a clinical trial. J Am Acad Dermatol 2019;80:1013–21.
72. Chen YL, Gutowska-Owsiak D, Hardman CS, et al. Proof-of-concept clinical trial of etokimab shows a key role for IL-33 in atopic dermatitis pathogenesis. Sci Transl Med 2019;11(515):eaax2945.
73. Guttman-Yassky E, Pavel AB, Zhou L, et al. GBR 830, an anti-OX40, improves skin gene signatures and clinical scores in patients with atopic dermatitis. J Allergy Clin Immunol 2019;144:482–93.e7.
74. Gittler JK, Shemer A, Suárez-Fariñas M, et al. Progressive activation of T(H)2/T(H)22 cytokines and selective epidermal proteins characterizes acute and chronic atopic dermatitis. J Allergy Clin Immunol 2012;130:1344–54.
75. Guttman-Yassky E, Brunner PM, Neumann AU, et al. Efficacy and safety of fezakinumab (an IL-22 monoclonal antibody) in adults with moderate-to-severe atopic dermatitis inadequately controlled by conventional treatments: A randomized, double-blind, phase 2a trial. J Am Acad Dermatol 2018;78:872–81.e6.
76. Brunner PM, Pavel AB, Khattri S, et al. Baseline IL-22 expression in patients with atopic dermatitis stratifies tissue responses to fezakinumab. J Allergy Clin Immunol 2019;143:142–54.

Current and Potential Biologic Drugs for the Treatment of Chronic Urticaria

Mario Sánchez-Borges, MD[a,b,*], Sandra González Díaz, MD[c,d],
Jose Antonio Ortega-Martell, MD[e], Maria Isabel Rojo, MD[f],
Ignacio J. Ansotegui, MD, PhD[g]

KEYWORDS

- Angioedema • Biologics • Chronic urticaria • Omalizumab

KEY POINTS

- Monoclonal anti–immunoglobulin E (omalizumab) is effective in a large proportion of patients with severe and refractory chronic spontaneous urticaria.
- Additional biologic medications designed to interfere with various inflammatory pathways involved in the pathogenesis of chronic urticaria are currently under investigation.
- Advances in the understanding of the mechanisms leading to chronic spontaneous urticaria will result in more efficacious and safe therapies for this complex disease in the near future.

INTRODUCTION

Chronic spontaneous (idiopathic) urticaria (CSU), defined as the occurrence of wheals, angioedema, or both for more than 6 weeks, affects 1% to 2% of the population.[1] It is more prevalent in women, and represents an important burden that compromises patients' quality of life, interferes with routine daily activities,[2] and frequently is associated with psychiatric comorbidities (depression and/or anxiety).[3] Mean yearly direct

Financial support: Author's funds.

[a] Allergy and Clinical Immunology Department, Centro Médico Docente La Trinidad, Caracas, Venezuela; [b] Allergy and Clinical Immunology Department, Clínica El Avila, Caracas, Venezuela; [c] Centro Regional de Excelencia CONACYT/WAO en Alergia Asma e Inmunologia Clínica, Hospital Universitario, Facultad de Medicina, Universidad Autonoma de Nuevo Leon, Monterrey, Nuevo León, Mexico; [d] San Francisco Centro de Especialistas Médicos 27196008(82); [e] Universidad Autónoma del Estado de Hidalgo, Artículo 27 # 102. Col. Constitución, Pachuca, Hidalgo CP 42080, Mexico; [f] Allergy Service, Juarez Hospital, Mexico City, Mexico; [g] Department of Allergy and Immunology, Hospital Quironsalud Bizkaia, Carretera Leioa-Unbe 33 bis, Erandio-Bilbao 48950, Spain
* Corresponding author. Clínica El Avila, 6a transversal Urb. Altamira, piso 8, consultorio 803, Caracas 1060, Venezuela.
E-mail address: sanchezbmario@gmail.com

and indirect costs of CSU in the United States have been estimated to be $244 million, with medication costs accounting for 62.5% and work absenteeism for 15.7% of the expenses.[4]

Although the mechanisms leading to CSU are not completely understood, important pathophysiologic advances have been accomplished in recent years. In general, it is thought that CSU is a chronic inflammatory skin disease in which various inflammatory cells and mediators are involved. This knowledge has permitted precision and personalized approaches to be envisioned for the management of this complex disease. As investigators discern immunologic pathways involved in the pathogenesis of CSU, novel therapeutic agents directed to specific molecular targets are being proposed.

According to the international guidelines for the definition, classification, diagnosis and management of urticaria,[5] the treatment of CSU is based on a first line consisting of nonsedating anti-H1 antihistamines at recommended doses. If no improvement is observed, the recommendation is to increase antihistamine dose up to 4 times. However, up to 50% of patients with CSU are not controlled with antihistamines.[6]

In patients unresponsive to antihistamines, add-on therapy with omalizumab is indicated, and alternatively cyclosporine could be administered to patients who do not respond to anti–immunoglobulin (Ig) E or in cases where this medication is not available, although this immunosuppressor has a less favorable profile of adverse effects than omalizumab.

Longer disease duration, higher severity, female gender, presence of angioedema, association of CSU with inducible urticaria, a positive autologous serum skin test, older age, nonsteroidal antiinflammatory drug hypersensitivity, and hypertension have been proposed as negative clinical prognostic factors in chronic urticaria (CU).[7,8] Laboratory markers of worse prognosis and increased severity are high levels of inflammatory markers (interleukin [IL]-6, IL-6sR, sgp130, IL-18, MMP, C-reactive protein, D-dimer, prothrombin fragments 1 + 2), low vitamin D levels, high mean platelet volume (MPV), basopenia, and cluster of differentiation (CD) 203c–positive basophil level[7] (Table 1).

This article reviews current therapy for CSU giving special attention to the use of biologic medications in patients with severe and refractory disease, including monoclonal anti-IgE antibodies (omalizumab) and various biologics that are under investigation and are directed to other potential targets involved in CSU.

Table 1
Prognostic biomarkers that have been proposed for chronic spontaneous urticaria

Clinical Markers	Laboratory Markers
• Longer disease duration	• Positive autologous serum skin test
• Higher severity	• IL-6
• Female gender	• IL-6sR
• Concomitant angioedema	• sgp130
• Association of CSU with inducible urticaria	• IL-18
	• C-reactive protein
• Older age	• MMP
• Nonsteroidal antiinflammatory drug hypersensitivity	• D-dimer
	• Prothrombin fragments 1 + 2
• Hypertension	• Low vitamin D levels,
	• High MPV
	• Basopenia
	• CD203c-positive basophils

PATHOGENESIS OF CHRONIC SPONTANEOUS URTICARIA

As already mentioned, the mechanisms underlying the origins of CSU have not been completely identified. It is widely recognized that mast cells are the key cellular elements involved in the production of all forms of urticaria and angioedema. Mast cell activation in response to various stimuli results in the release of inflammatory mediators in the skin that are able to induce the characteristic wheals and angioedema. Among those mediators, histamine, cysteinyl leukotrienes, prostaglandins, platelet-activating factor, cytokines, and chemokines induce sensory nerve stimulation (leading to pruritus), vasodilatation and plasma extravasation (leading to wheals and edema), and inflammatory cell recruitment. Also, upregulation of cell adhesion molecules in the endothelium; the release of neuropeptides and growth factors; and a mixed non-necrotizing inflammatory perivascular infiltrate of neutrophils, eosinophils, basophils, macrophages, and CD4+ T lymphocytes are present.

In the skin of patients with CU, there is an increase of mast cell numbers and releasability, basophil abnormalities (basopenia; altered FcεRI function; increased levels of IL-31, which stimulates basophil chemotaxis and activates IL-4 and IL-13 release; increased expression of CD63), and activation of the coagulation cascade. Hypersensitivity to sweat substances has been proposed as a mechanism of cholinergic urticaria,[9] whereas various infectious agents (*Helicobacter pylori*, human herpesvirus-6, *Blastocystis hominis*, *Toxocara*, *Anisakis simplex*) have been suggested by some investigators as triggers of CU.

Skin mast cells can be activated by multiple pathways, including the following (**Table 2**):

Table 2
Putative mast cell/basophil activation pathways in chronic urticarial

Receptors	Agonists	Mechanism
Immunoglobulin Receptors		
FcεRI/FcεRII	Allergen-specific IgE	Allergy
	Autoantigen-specific IgE	Autoimmunity type I
	IgE-specific IgG	Autoimmunity type IIb
	FcεRI-specific IgG	Autoimmunity type IIb
FcγRII	Autoantigen-specific IgG	Autoimmunity type IIb
Toll-like Receptors		
Toll-like receptor	PAMPs	Infection
	DAMPs	Inflammation
G Protein–coupled Receptors		
PAR2	Tryptase	Inflammation
	Thrombin	Coagulation cascade
C3aR/C5aR	C3a, CSa	Complement cascade
MRGPRX2	Neuropeptides	Neurogenic inflammation
	Cysteine proteases	Inflammation
	Antimicrobial peptides	Infection
	Cationic proteins	Eosinophilic inflammation
	Fluoroquinolones	Non-IgE anaphylaxis
	Vancomycin	Red-man syndrome
	Morphine, atracurium	Perioperative anaphylaxis

Abbreviations: DAMPs, damage-associated molecular patterns; PAMPs, pathogen-associated molecular patterns.

1. Allergen-specific IgE binding to allergen and to high-affinity receptors (FcɛRI) on the mast cell membrane. This mechanism is commonly present in acute urticaria (eg, urticaria induced by penicillin or food allergens) but rarely participates in CU.
2. Autoimmunity: various autoimmune mechanisms have been shown in CU; for example, autoreactive IgG antibodies directed to FcɛRI or to IgE, autoantibodies to autoallergens (thyroid antigens, DNA, IL-24). Type I autoimmunity (autoallergy) is caused by IgE versus autoantigens, whereas type II autoimmunity is related to IgG to FcɛRI, to FcɛRII, or to IgE. These autoantibodies are complement-fixing IgG1 and IgG3 immunoglobulins, which induce the release of C5a. Chronic spontaneous urticaria is often associated with other autoimmune diseases, including autoimmune thyroiditis, celiac disease, Sjögren syndrome, systemic lupus erythematosus, rheumatoid arthritis, and type 1 diabetes. In addition, CD4+ T cells recognizing the FcɛRI have recently been recognized.[10]
3. Complement-dependent basophil activation: as proposed in urticaria induced by radiocontrast media.[11,12]
4. Mas-related G protein–coupled receptor X2 (MGRPRx2), a novel mast cell receptor that can be activated by different ligands such as neuropeptides, cysteine proteases, antimicrobial peptides, cationic proteins released from activated eosinophils[13] and human β-defensins.[14] It has been shown that this mast cell receptor is upregulated in the skin from patients with severe CSU.
5. Histamine-releasing factors (HRFs): for example, translationally controlled tumor factor (TCTP) and other HRFs have been proposed as mast cell activators in CU. Dimeric TCTP promotes mast cell and basophil degranulation.[15]
6. Activation of the coagulation system by tissue factor leading to thrombin generation that is able to induce mast cell degranulation (**Fig. 1**).

BIOLOGIC MEDICATIONS FOR CHRONIC SPONTANEOUS URTICARIA

At present, omalizumab is the only biologic drug approved by regulatory agencies as add-on therapy for the treatment of adult and adolescent patients (aged $\geq$ 12 years) with CSU who remain symptomatic despite optimized H1-antihistamine therapy. In addition, there are several other biologics that have been proposed, used off license, or are being investigated for severe CSU, including ligelizumab, quilizumab, intravenous immunoglobulin (IVIg), tumor necrosis factor alpha (TNF-α) inhibitors, anti-CD20 (rituximab), IL-1 inhibitors, Syk inhibitors, PGDR2 antagonists, Btk inhibitors, and anti–Siglec-8.

Anti–Immunoglobulin E: Omalizumab, Ligelizumab, Quilizumab

Omalizumab
For many years, it was thought that IgE was not a major factor involved in the pathogenesis of CU. This concept was challenged by the demonstration of clinical efficacy of a monoclonal anti-IgE antibody in patients with refractory CSU.[16] Anti-IgE monoclonal antibody (omalizumab) was the first biologic agent licensed for the treatment of CSU refractory to antihistamines. In double-blinded placebo-controlled studies, about 40% of patients showed a complete response and 50% to 70% a partial response to this therapy.[17–19] These effectiveness results have been confirmed through meta-analysis.[20]

Recommended doses of 150 mg and 300 mg are given subcutaneously every 4 weeks. In some patients, a delayed response of up to 6 months is observed, although many patients experience relapses of CU after discontinuing the treatment, whereas retreatment generally induces a rapid symptom remission. Although there are

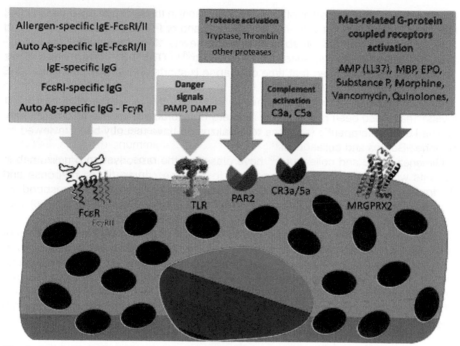

Fig. 1. Selected pathways of mast cell activation putatively involved in chronic urticaria. AMP, antimicrobial peptide; DAMP, damage-associated molecular pattern; EPO, erythropoietin; MBP, major basic protein; PAMP, pathogen-associated molecular pattern; TLR, toll-like receptor.

no controlled studies, there is evidence from case reports and small series showing that omalizumab may be also effective in inducible urticarias.[21]

Regarding the main mechanisms of action, omalizumab binding to soluble IgE and a decrease of FcεRI receptors on skin mast cell membrane have been proposed.[22] Additional mechanisms of action that have been suggested are summarized in **Box 1**.

A positive basophil histamine release assay (BHRA) and autologous serum skin test seem to correlate with a slow response to omalizumab,[23] whereas higher levels of FcεRI expression predict a faster response.[24] The lack of basophil CD203c-

Box 1
Mechanisms of action of omalizumab in chronic urticaria
Reduction of IgE levels
Dissociation of the IgE-FcεRI binding
Reduction of IgE receptors on mast cells and basophils
Reduction of mast cell/basophil degranulation
Reversion of basopenia and improvement of the IgE receptor function in basophils
Reduction of anti-FcεRI and anti-IgE IgG autoantibody activity
Reduction of antiautoantigen IgE autoantibodies

upregulating activlty (a marker of basophil activation) in the serum of patients with CU, reflecting the presence of autoantibodies to IgE and/or FcεRI, correlated with a good clinical response to omalizumab.[25] Also, higher levels of total serum IgE are associated with greater responsiveness to omalizumab[26,27] (**Table 3**). Nevertheless, Ertas and colleagues[28] observed that time of relapse is shorter in patients with serum IgE level higher than 100 kU/L.

The reduction of plasmatic D-dimer levels[29] and the reduction of serum IL-31 levels[30] have also been proposed as markers of favorable response to omalizumab. Biomarkers of therapeutic response to omalizumab have recently been reviewed by Sánchez-Borges and colleagues.[31]

Gimenez Arnau and colleagues[32] have classified the responses to omalizumab in patients with CSU in 5 profiles according to the time course of the response and the improvement in the Urticaria Activity Score 7 (UAS7) as follows: fast responders, slow responders, complete responders (UAS7 = 0), good responders (UAS7 1–6), partial responders (UAS7 7–15), and nonresponders (UAS7 >16).

Although omalizumab is efficacious in a many patients with severe CU, there are some issues that interfere with its wider use, mainly its high cost, the frequent occurrence of disease relapses once the treatment is suspended, and the observation that the optimal duration of the treatment has not been established.[33] Anaphylaxis triggered by omalizumab in patients with CU seems to be infrequent, although the rate of anaphylaxis in patients with moderate to severe asthma receiving omalizumab has been estimated to be approximately 1 in 1000.[34]

Ligelizumab

Ligelizumab is an IgG1κ high-affinity humanized monoclonal anti-IgE antibody that binds with higher affinity to the Cε3 domain of IgE than omalizumab, with a 6-fold to 9-fold greater suppression of allergen-induced skin prick tests in vivo. The dissociation constant (Kd) of omalizumab is 6 to 8 nM, whereas for ligelizumab it is 139 pM.

In a phase 2b trial, patients with CU received ligelizumab at a dose of 24 mg, 72 mg, or 240 mg; omalizumab at a dose of 300 mg; or placebo subcutaneously every 4 weeks for 20 weeks, or a single 120-mg dose of ligelizumab. Three-hundred and eighty-two patients were randomized, and, at week 12, 30%, 51%, and 42% of patients treated with 24 mg, 72 mg, and 240 mg had complete control of hives, compared with 26% in the omalizumab group and 0% in the placebo group. No safety concerns were apparent in this study.[35] Ligelizumab showed dose-dependent and time-dependent suppression of free IgE, basophil FcεRI, and basophil surface IgE superior in extent

Table 3	
Biomarkers of response to omalizumab in chronic urticaria	
Biomarkers	**Response**
BHRA	Slow response
Positive autologous serum skin test	Slow response
Higher levels of FcεRI expression	Faster response
Lack of basophil CD203c-upregulating activity (a marker of basophil activation) in the serum	Good clinical response
Higher levels of total serum IgE	Greater responsiveness
Reduction of plasmatic D-dimer levels	Favorable response
Reduction of serum IL-31 levels	Favorable response

(free IgE and surface IgE) and duration to omalizumab. Skin prick wheal responses to allergen were suppressed by greater than 95% and 41% in subjects treated subcutaneously with ligelizumab or omalizumab, respectively.[36] A reduction was observed in weekly rescue medication use early in the core study with ligelizumab treatment compared with placebo through week 20, whereas ligelizumab 240 mg induced a sustained decrease of rescue medication use in a 1-year extension study.[37] In the same core study, at week 12, 87.5% and 94.9% of patients treated with ligelizumab 72 mg and 240 mg were angioedema free, respectively, versus 76.3% for omalizumab and 68.3% for placebo.[38]

Quilizumab

Quilizumab is a humanized monoclonal antibody that targets the M1 prime segment of membrane-expressed IgE on IgE-switched B cells and plasmablasts. By causing the depletion of IgE-switched B cells and plasmablasts, it reduces serum IgE levels.

In a multicenter, double-blind study in 32 adult patients with CSU who were symptomatic despite H1 antihistamine treatment with or without leukotriene receptor antagonists and received placebo or quilizumab 450 mg via subcutaneous route at days 1 and 29, the absolute change at week 20 in the weekly itch score decreased by 3.3 points and 1.5 points in patients treated with quilizumab relative to the placebo group at weeks 4 and 20, respectively, a difference that was not statistically significant. Quilizumab reduced median serum total IgE level only by approximately 30% from baseline at week 20.[39]

OTHER BIOLOGICS POTENTIALLY USEFUL FOR THE TREATMENT OF CHRONIC URTICARIA

The following biologics have been proposed for therapy for CU: IVIg, TNF-alpha inhibitors, IL-1 inhibitors, anti-CD20, anti–Siglec-8, anti–thymic stromal lymphopoietin (TSLP), anti–IL-4Rα, anti–IL-5, anti–IL-5Rα, and anti–IL-13. Some of them have been used off label in case reports or small series of patients, and others are currently under investigation in phase 2 (**Table 4**).

Intravenous Immunoglobulins

IVIg prepared by pooling plasma from healthy donors has been used for the treatment of CSU, as is done in other autoimmune diseases. However, only uncontrolled case series are reported in the literature regarding this modality of therapy. High-dose IVIg induced significant improvement of severe autoimmune urticaria in 9 out of 10 patients,[40] as well as in 5 out of 8 patients with severe unremitting delayed-pressure urticaria (DPU)[41] and in 5 out of 6 patients with therapy-resistant CSU.[42]

Low-dose IVIg induced clinical improvement in 26 out of 28 patients with severe autoimmune CU refractory to conventional treatment.[43] Mechanisms of action of IVIg in CU might be based on Fc receptor blockade, increase of FcγRIIB expression, effects of antiidiotypic antibodies, modulation of cytokines, enhancement of regulatory T-cell function, and accelerated clearance of autoantibodies.[44–46] IVIg has also been shown to be effective in solar urticaria.[47]

It has been proposed that IVIg could be used as an alternative treatment in omalizumab nonresponder patients.[48] However, 2 studies showed that a single cycle (2 g/kg) of IVIg is unlikely to induce sustained remission of CU.[49,50] In the 2009 European Academy of Allergy, Asthma and Immunology (EAACI)/Global Allergy and Asthma European Network (GA2LEN)/EDF/ World Allergy Organization (WAO) guidelines, IVIg is recommended only as a last option to be applied in centers specialized in CSU.[51] Side effects of IVIg include flushing, myalgia, headache, fever, chills, nausea,

Table 4
Biologics with potential usefulness in chronic urticaria

Biologic	Remarks
IVIg	Potentially useful in severe autoimmune and delayed-pressure urticaria. Cost and the need for intravenous route limit its use
TNF-α inhibitors (etanercept, adalimumab, infliximab)	Some benefit reported in refractory CSU and delayed-pressure urticaria. Risk of serious adverse effects
IL-1 inhibitors (anakinra, canakinumab)	Potentially useful in Schnitzler, syndrome, cryopyrin-associated periodic syndrome, delayed-pressure urticaria, cold urticaria, and urticarial vasculitis
Anti-CD20 (rituximab)	Efficacious in isolated cases of autoimmune urticaria and idiopathic angioedema
Anti–Siglec-8 (AK002)	Induced improvement of uncontrolled CU, symptomatic dermographism and cholinergic urticaria
Anti-TSLP (tezepelumab)	No data available
Anti–IL-4Rα (dupilumab)	Little information available at this time
Anti–IL-5/IL-5Rα (mepolizumab, reslizumab, benralizumab)	No data available
Anti–IL-13 (antukizumab, lebrikizumab, tralokinumab)	No data available

vomiting, chest tightness, wheezing, abnormal blood pressure, tachycardia, and aseptic meningitis. High cost and the need for intravenous access limit the use of this therapeutic approach.

Tumor Necrosis Factor Alpha Inhibitors

TNF-α is upregulated in skin and serum in patients with urticaria[52,53] and may play a role in the pathogenesis of some cases of CU. Etanercept, adalimumab, and infliximab have been used in patients with CU and urticarial vasculitis.

A study showed that 60% of patients with refractory CU responded to etanercept 50 mg weekly or adalimumab 40 mg twice monthly. Fifteen percent showed partial response and 25% did not respond. Sand and Thomsen[54] reported complete or almost complete resolution of CU in 12 out of 20 patients and partial response in 3 additional patients with adalimumab (16 patients treated) or etanercept (4 patients treated).

Anti-TNF treatment is recommended in the international urticaria guidelines only as a last option for DPU.[51] Etanercept, a competitive inhibitor of TNF-α, at a dose of 25 mg twice weekly induced rapid and complete improvement of DPU in a 42-year-old patient with psoriasis and concomitant DPU who remained free of urticaria or angioedema even after switching to infliximab,[55] and Bingsgaard and colleagues[56] reported the beneficial effects of the TNF-α inhibitor adalimumab in 6 out of 8 patients with recalcitrant CU.

Various investigators have suggested the use of TNF-α inhibitors in patients with antihistamine-refractory CSU who do not respond to or do not tolerate omalizumab. Wilson and colleagues[57] treated 6 patients with refractory CU (4 with etanercept, 1 with adalimumab, and 1 with infliximab) and observed improvement in all of them.

When considering the indication of TNF-α inhibitors in patients with CSU, increased risk of serious infections, lymphoma, and other malignancies must be taken into account.

Interleukin-1 Inhibitors: Anakinra, Canakinumab

Anakinra is a recombinant human IL-1 receptor antagonist that inhibits IL-1 binding to its IL-1 type I receptor (IL-R1).[58] Canakinumab is a fully human anti–IL-1β monoclonal antibody that selectively blocks IL-1β and has no cross reactivity with other IL-1 family members, including IL-1α and IL-1Ra.

Schnitzler syndrome is a disorder caused by an IgM or IgG monoclonal gammopathy that is characterized by nonpruritic urticarial rash, intermittent fever, myalgias, bone pain, increased erythrocyte sedimentation rate, lymphadenopathy, and monoclonal IgM.[59] IL-1 seems to play a critical role in the disease, because it responds to anakinra. In 29 patients with Schnitzler syndrome treated with anakinra, 83% achieved complete remission and 17% partial remission, although 3 patients developed neutropenia and 6 severe infections.[60] In a randomized placebo-controlled study, canakinumab induced complete responses in 5 out of 7 patients with Schnitzler syndrome, whereas responses to placebo were observed in 0 out of 13 patients.[61] A patient with CU, polyarthritis, and polyclonal IgA resembling Schnitzler syndrome experienced rapid resolution of the urticarial rash and arthritis after receiving daily anakinra,[62] and another patient with CU associated with polyclonal IgG and IgA also responded to anakinra.[63]

In the IL-1β–mediated autoinflammatory diseases cryopyrin-associated periodic syndrome and Schnitzler syndrome, a nonitchy urticarial rash is present. Various reports have observed the improvement of urticarial rashes induced by IL-1–blocking therapies in those autoinflammatory syndromes[64,65] as well as in DPU and cold urticaria.[66,67] Isolated cases of urticarial vasculitis responding to canakinumab and anakinra have been published. Patients showed increased levels of IL-1R and IL-6, which decreased after IL-1 blockade.[68,69]

Remission of urticarial vasculitis with a 300-mg single dose of anakinra in 10 patients in an open-label study was reported by Venzor and colleagues,[70] with significant reductions in mean total urticarial vasculitis activity score, global disease activity, and physician-based mean visual analogue scale (VAS) at day 14, patient-reported VAS, reduction of inflammatory markers, and improvement of quality of life, whereas the treatment was well tolerated. More common adverse effects of IL-1 inhibitors are respiratory tract infections, gastrointestinal symptoms, and hypertension.

Anti-CD20: Rituximab

Rituximab, a chimeric murine/human recombinant monoclonal antibody directed against CD20, inhibits autoantibody production by depleting memory B lymphocytes. Although no randomized blinded trials have been performed, it was effective in 3 patients with autoimmune urticaria,[71–73] but was ineffective in another.[74] It was also effective in a 19-year-old woman with severe steroid-dependent idiopathic angioedema.[75]

Some investigators have suggested that rituximab may be an option in very resistant autoimmune urticaria, although side effects, including fatigue, arthralgias, and swelling around the infusion site, may limit its usefulness.[76] No studies on the effects of other anti-CD20 antibodies (ofatumumab, ocrelizumab) in patients with CU are available.

Anti–Siglec-8

Siglecs (sialic acid immunoglobulinlike lectins) are members of the immunoglobulin gene family that contain sialoside-binding N-terminal domains. They are cell surface proteins found predominantly on the membranes of cells of the immune system. Siglec-8 is selectively expressed on human eosinophils and mast cells, and weakly on basophils.[77]

AK002 is an anti–Siglec-8 antibody that selectively inhibits mast cells and depletes eosinophils. In a phase 2a open-label study in patients with uncontrolled CU despite treatment with anti-H1 antihistamines, substantial improvements in UAS7 were reported, and 90% were responders according to the Urticaria Control Test, whereas, in refractory patients, 86% responded. Eighty-two percent of patients with cholinergic urticaria and 70% of patients with symptomatic dermographism also responded. The treatment was well tolerated, and the most common adverse effects were mild/moderate infusion-related reactions (flushing, feeling of warmth, headache, nausea, or dizziness).[78]

Anti–thymic Stromal Lymphopoietin

TSLP is a TH2-initiating cytokine that activates mast cells by innate immune mechanisms and is increased in lesional skin of patients with CSU.[79] A human monoclonal IgG2κ antibody that blocks the interaction of TSLP with its receptor (AMG157) could be a therapeutic option to treat CSU.

Anti–interleukin-4Rα: dupilumab

Dupilumab, an anti–IL-4Rα monoclonal antibody that blocks actions of IL-4 and IL-13, may be a valuable treatment of CSU resistant to other therapies. Lee and Simpson[80] reported 1 patient with CSU unresponsive to omalizumab 600 mg, antihistamines, and prednisone in which dupilumab was effective. A possible mechanism of action of dupilumab could be the blockade of the induction of B cell to plasma cell subclass switching from IgM to IgE and limitation of the IL-13 inflammatory cascade that leads to pruritus in CSU.

Anti–interleukin-5 and anti–interleukin-5Rα: mepolizumab, reslizumab, benralizumab

Increased numbers of eosinophils have been observed in nonlesional skin of patients with CSU, and increased IL-5 levels are present in CSU skin lesions.[79,81] It has been proposed that tissue factor released by eosinophils can induce the activation of coagulation cascade, resulting in thrombin generation, which can increase vascular permeability by inducing degranulation of mast cells.[82]

Biologics interfering with IL-5 (anti–IL-5 monoclonal antibodies mepolizumab and reslizumab) and its receptor (benralizumab, an anti–IL-5-Rα) are potential therapies for CSU, although currently not enough data supporting this concept are available.[83,84]

Anti–interleukin-13: antukizumab, lebrikizumab, tralokinumab

Increased levels of IL-13 are present in patients with CSU.[85,86] However, no studies on the treatment of CU with anti–IL-13 monoclonal antibodies have been reported.

ADDITIONAL THERAPEUTIC TARGETS

There are several other inflammatory pathways that could be targeted for the treatment of CU, although currently there are no published studies on these potential approaches. They include Syk inhibitors (GSK 2646264), PGDR2/CRTh2 antagonists

(AZD1981), Btk inhibitors (GDC-0853), β7 integrins (RhuMabβ7), α4 integrins (natalizumab), and α4β7 integrins (vedolizumab).

SUMMARY

The only currently approved biologic treatment of severe and refractory CU is omalizumab, a monoclonal anti-IgE antibody. Controlled studies have shown that it is effective and safe in a significant proportion of patients with severe CU. In patients who do not respond to omalizumab, cyclosporine constitutes an alternative, although its toxicity requires that it is applied under close monitoring by physicians experienced in its use. The high-affinity humanized monoclonal anti-IgE antibody, ligelizumab, showed higher affinity than omalizumab and it is effective at lower doses. Several other biologics that are potentially useful for CSU are discussed in this article.

CLINICS CARE POINTS

- The pathogenesis of CSU is complex, and probably various pathways may result in the production of wheals and angioedema.
- Omalizumab is the only biologic medication currently approved by regulatory agencies for patients with CSU who do not respond to nonsedating antihistamines.
- Because of patient phenotype heterogeneity, the duration of omazulimab treatment in patients with CSU has not been established.
- Biomarkers for diagnosis, prognosis, and therapeutic response to guideline-recommended medications are pending validation.
- New biologics targeting key receptors, cytokines, and other mediators are being actively investigated and it is expected, that in the near future, physicians will use more efficacious and safe biologic drugs to treat patients with refractory CSU.

CONFLICTS OF INTEREST

M. Sánchez-Borges has received honoraria for lectures from Novartis. S.G. Díaz, J.A. Ortega-Martell, M.I. Rojo, and I.J. Ansotegui have nothing to disclose.

REFERENCES

1. Zuberbier T, Balke M, Worm M, et al. Epidemiology of urticaria: A representative cross-sectional population survey. Clin Exp Dermatol 2010;35:869–73.
2. Baiardini I, Giardini A, Pasquali M, et al. Quality of life and patient's satisfaction in chronic urticaria and respiratory allergy. Allergy 2003;58:621–3.
3. Staubach P, Eckhardt-Henn A, Dechene M, et al. Quality of life in patients with chronic urticaria is differentially impaired and determined by psychiatric comorbidity. Br J Dermatol 2006;154:294–8.
4. Delong LK, Culler SD, Saini SS, et al. Annual direct and indirect health care costs of chronic idiopathic urticaria: A cost analysis of 50 nonimmunosuppressed patients. Arch Dermatol 2008;144:35–9.
5. Zuberbier T, Aberer W, Asero R, et al. The EAACI/GA2LEN/EDF/WAO Guideline for the definition, classification, diagnosis and management of urticaria. Allergy 2018;73:1393–414.
6. Kaplan AP. Treatment of chronic spontaneous urticaria. Allergy Asthma Immunol Res 2012;4:326–31.
7. Folci M, Heffler E, Canonica GW, et al. Cutting edge: Biomarkers for chronic spontaneous urticaria. J Immunol Res 2018;2018:5615109.

8. Sánchez-Borges M, Caballero-Fonseca F, Capriles-Hulett A, et al. Factors linked to disease severity and time to remission in patients with chronic spontaneous urticaria. J Eur Acad Dermatol Venereol 2017;31:964–71.

9. Takahagi S, Tanaka A, Hide M. Sweat allergy. Allergol Int 2018;67:435–41.

10. Auyeung P, Mittag D, Hodgkin PD, et al. Autoreactive T cells in chronic spontaneous urticaria target the IgE Fc receptor Iα subunit. J Allergy Clin Immunol 2016;138:761–8.

11. Kikuchi Y, Kaplan AP. A role for C5a in augmenting IgG-dependent histamine release from basophils in chronic urticaria. Pathogenesis of chronic urticaria. J Allergy Clin Immunol 2002;109:114–8.

12. Kaplan AP, Greaves M. Pathogenesis of Chronic Urticaria. Clin Exp Allergy 2009; 39:777–87.

13. Fujisawa D, Kashiwakura J, Kita H, et al. Expression of Mas-related gene X2 on mast cells is upregulated in the skin of patients with severe chronic urticaria. J Allergy Clin Immunol 2014;134:622–33.

14. Subramanian H, Gupta K, Ali H. Roles of Mas-related G protein-coupled receptor X2 on mast cell-mediated host defense, pseudoallergic drug reactions, and chronic inflammatory diseases. J Allergy Clin Immunol 2016;138:700–10.

15. Ulambayar B, Lee H, Yang EM, et al. Dimerized, Not Monomeric, Translationally Controlled Tumor Protein Induces Basophil Activation and Mast Cell Degranulation in Chronic Urticaria. Immune Netw 2019;19:e20.

16. Sánchez-Borges M, Capriles-Hulett A, Caballero-Fonseca F, et al. Justification for IgE as a therapeutic target in chronic spontaneous urticaria. Eur Ann Allergy Clin Immunol 2017;49:148–53.

17. Kaplan A, Ledford D, Ashby M, et al. Omalizumab in patients with symptomatic chronic idiopathic/spontaneous urticaria despite standard combination therapy. J Allergy Clin Immunol 2013;132:101–9.

18. Maurer M, Rosen K, Hsieh HJ, et al. Omalizumab for the treatment of chronic idiopathic or spontaneous urticaria. N Engl J Med 2013;368:924–35.

19. Saini SS, Bindslev-Jensen C, Maurer M, et al. Efficacy and safety of omalizumab in patients with chronic idiopathic/spontaneous urticaria who remain symptomatic on H1 antihistamines: A randomized, placebo-controlled study. J Invest Dermatol 2015;135:67–75.

20. Zhao ZT, Ji CM, Yu WJ, et al. Omalizumab for the treatment of chronic spontaneous urticaria: A meta-analysis of randomized clinical trials. J Allergy Clin Immunol 2016;137:1742–50.

21. Maurer M, Altrichter S, Schmetzer O, et al. Immunoglobulin E-mediated autoimmunity. Front Immunol 2018;9:689.

22. Metz M, Staubach P, Bauer A, et al. Clinical efficacy of omalizumab in chronic spontaneous urticaria is associated with a reduction of FcεRI-positive cells in the skin. Theranostics 2017;7:1266–76.

23. Konstantinou GN, Asero R, Maurer M, et al. EAACI/GA2LEN task force consensus report: The autologous serum skin test in urticaria. Allergy 2009;64:1256–68.

24. Deza G, Bertolin-Colilla M, Sánchez S, et al. Basophil FcεRI expression is linked to time to omalizumab response in chronic spontaneous urticaria. J Allergy Clin Immunol 2018;141:2313–6.

25. Yasnowsky K, Dreskin S, Efan B, et al. Chronic urticaria sera increase basophil CD203c expression. J Allergy Clin Immunol 2006;117:1430–4.

26. Straesser MD, Oliver E, Palacios T, et al. Serum IgE as an immunological marker to predict response to omalizumab treatment in symptomatic chronic urticaria. J Allergy Clin Immunol Pract 2017;6:1386–8.

27. Viswanathan RK, Moss MH, Mathur SK. Retrospective analysis of the efficacy of omalizumab in chronic refractory urticaria. Allergy Asthma Proc 2013;34:446–52.
28. Ertas R, Ozyurt K, Ozlu EJ, et al. Increased IgE levels are linked to faster relapse in patients with omalizumab-discontinued chronic spontaneous urticaria. J Allergy Clin Immunol 2017;140:1749–51.
29. Asero R, Marzano AV, Cugno M. D-dimer plasma levels parallel the clinical response to omalizumab in patients with severe chronic spontaneous urticaria. Int Arch Allergy Immunol 2017;172:40–4.
30. Altrichter S, Hawro T, Hänel K, et al. Successful omalizumab treatment in chronic spontaneous urticaria is associated with lowering of serum IL-31 levels. J Eur Acad Dermatol Venereol 2016;30:454–5.
31. Sánchez-Borges M, Capriles-Hulett A, Caballero-Fonseca F, et al. Biomarkers of treatment efficacy in patients with chronic spontaneous urticaria. Eur Ann Allergy Clin Immunol 2018;50:5–9.
32. Gimenez Arnau AM, Valero Santiago A, Bartra Tomás J. Therapeutic Strategy According to Differences in Response to Omalizumab in Patients With Chronic Spontaneous Urticaria. J Investig Allergol Clin Immunol 2019;29:338–48.
33. Incorvaia C, Mauro M, Makri E, et al. Two decades with omalizumab: What we still have to learn. Biologics 2018;12:135–42.
34. Bernstein JA, Lang DM, Khan D, et al. The diagnosis and management of acute and chronic urticaria: 2014 update. J Allergy Clin Immunol 2014;133:1270–7.
35. Maurer M, Gimenez-Arnau AM, Sussman G, et al. Ligelizumab for chronic spontaneous urticaria. N Engl J Med 2019;381:1321–32.
36. Arm JP, Bottoli L, Skerjanee A, et al. Pharmacokinetics, pharmacodynamics and safety of QGE031 (Ligelizumab), a novel high-affinity anti-IgE antibody, in atopic subjects. Clin Exp Allergy 2014;44:1371–85.
37. Sitz K, Soong W, Lanier B, et al. Ligelizumab reduces rescue medication use in patients with chronic spontaneous urticaria: Phase 2B study results. Ann Allergy Asthma Immunol 2019;123:S28.
38. Soong W, Lanier B, Sitz K, et al. Ligelizumab achieves sustained control of angioedema in patients with chronic spontaneous urticaria. Ann Allergy Asthma Immunol 2019;123:S27.
39. Harris JM, Cabanski CR, Scheerens H, et al. A randomized trial of Quilizumab in adults with refractory chronic spontaneous urticaria. J Allergy Clin Immunol 2016;138:1730–2.
40. O'Donnell BF, Barr RM, Black AK, et al. Intravenous immunoglobulin in autoimmune chronic urticaria. Br J Dermatol 1998;138:101–6.
41. Dawn G, Urcelay M, Ah-Weng A, et al. Effect of high-dose intravenous immunoglobulin in delayed pressure urticaria. Br J Dermatol 2003;149:836–40.
42. Mitzel-Kaoukhov H, Staubach P, Müller-Brenne T. Effect of high-dose intravenous immunoglobulin treatment in therapy-resistant chronic spontaneous urticaria. Ann Allergy Asthma Immunol 2010;104:253–8.
43. Pereira C, Tavares B, Carrapatoso I, et al. Low-dose intravenous gammaglobulin in the treatment of severe autoimmune urticaria. Eur Ann Allergy Clin Immunol 2007;39:237–42.
44. Kroiss M, Landthaler M, Stolz W. The effectiveness of low-dose intravenous immunoglobulin in chronic urticaria. Acta Derm Venereol 2000;80:225.
45. Spellberg B. Mechanism of intravenous immune globulin therapy. N Engl J Med 1999;341:57–8.
46. Schwab I, Nimmerjahn F. Intravenous immunoglobulin therapy. How does IgG modulate the immune system? Nat Rev Immunol 2013;13:176–89.

47. Correia I, Silva J, Filipe P, et al. Solar urticaria treated successfully with intravenous high-dose immunoglobulin: A case report. Photodermatol Photoimmunol Photomed 2008;24:330–1.

48. Rutkowski K, Grattan CEH. How to manage chronic urticaria 'beyond' guidelines: A practical algorithm. Clin Exp Allergy 2017;47:710–8.

49. Hrabak T, Calabria CW. Multiple treatment cycles of high-dose intravenous immunoglobulin for chronic spontaneous urticaria. Ann Allergy Asthma Immunol 2010; 105:245–6.

50. Asero R. Are IVIg for chronic unremitting urticaria effective? Allergy 2000;55: 1099–101.

51. Zuberbier T, Asero R, Bindslev-Jensen C, et al. EAACI/GA(2)LEN/EDF/WAO guideline: management of urticaria. Allergy 2009;64:1427–43.

52. Hermes B, Prochazka AK, Haas N, et al. Upregulation of TNF-alpha and IL-3 expression in lesional and uninvolved skin in different types of urticaria. J Allergy Clin Immunol 1999;103:307–14.

53. Piconi S, Trabattoni D, Iemoli E, et al. Immune profiles of patients with chronic idiopathic urticaria. Int Arch Allergy Immunol 2002;128:59–66.

54. Sand FL, Thomsen SF. TNF-alpha inhibitors for chronic urticaria: Experience in 20 patients. J Allergy (Cairo) 2013;2013:130905.

55. Magerl M, Philipp S, Manasterski M, et al. Successful treatment of delayed pressure urticaria with anti-TNF-α. J Allergy Clin Immunol 2007;119:752–4.

56. Bingsgaard N, Skoy L, Zacharine C. Treatment of refractory chronic spontaneous urticaria with adalimumab. Acta Derm Venereol 2017;97:524–5.

57. Wilson LH, Eliason MJ, Leiferman KM, et al. Treatment of refractory chronic urticaria with tumor necrosis factor-alpha inhibitors. J Am Acad Dermatol 2011;64: 1221–2.

58. Hannum CH, Wilcox CJ, Arend WP, et al. Interleukin-1 receptor antagonist activity of a human interleukin-1 inhibitor. Nature 1990;343:336–40.

59. Simon A, Asli B, Braun-Falco M, et al. Schnitzler's syndrome: Diagnosis, treatment, and follow-up. Allergy 2013;68:562–8.

60. Neel A, Henry B, Barbarot S, et al. Long-term effectiveness and safety of interleukin-1 receptor antagonist (anakinra) in Schnitzler's syndrome: A French multicenter study. Autoimmun Rev 2014;13:1035–41.

61. Krause K, Tsianakas A, Wagner N, et al. Efficacy and safety of canakinumab in Schnitzler syndrome: A multicenter randomized placebo-controlled study. J Allergy Clin Immunol 2017;139:1311–20.

62. Cong-Qiu C. Chronic urticaria and arthritis with polyclonal IgA: Rapid response and clinical remission with interleukin 1 blockade. J Rheumatol 2010;37:881–2.

63. Treudler R, Kauer F, Simon JC. Striking effect of the IL-1 receptor antagonist Anakinra in chronic urticarial rash with polyclonal increase in IgG and IgA. Acta Derm Venereol 2007;87:280–1.

64. Schuster C, Kranke B, Aberer E, et al. Schnitzler syndrome: Response to Anakinra in two cases and review of the literature. Int J Dermatol 2009;48:1190–4.

65. Lachman HJ, Kone-Paul I, Kuemmerle-Deschner JB, et al. Use of Canakinumab in the Cryopirin-Associated Periodic Syndrome. N Engl J Med 2009;360:2416–25.

66. Lenormand C, Lipsker D. Efficiency of interleukin-1 blockade in refractory delayed pressure urticaria. Ann Intern Med 2012;157:599–600.

67. Bodar EJ, Simon A, De VIsser M, et al. Complete remission of severe idiopathic cold urticaria on interleukin-1 receptor antagonist (Anakinra). Neth J Med 2009; 67:302–5.

68. Krause K, Mahamed A, Weller K, et al. Efficacy and safety of Canakinumab in urticarial vasculitis: An open label study. J Allergy Clin Immunol 2013;132:751–4.
69. Botsios C, Seriso P, Punzi L, et al. Non-complementemic urticarial vasculitis: Successful treatment with the IL-1 receptor antagonist anakinra. Scand J Rheumatol 2007;36:236–7.
70. Venzor J, Lee WL, Huston DP. Urticarial vasculitis. Clin Rev Allergy Immunol 2002; 23:201–16.
71. Arkwright PD. Anti-CD20 or anti-IgE therapy for severe chronic autoimmune urticaria. J Allergy Clin Immunol 2009;123:510–1.
72. Chakravarty SD, Yee AF, Paget SA. Rituximab successfully treats refractory chronic autoimmune urticaria caused by IgE receptor autoantibodies. J Allergy Clin Immunol 2011;128:1354–5.
73. Steinweg SA, Gaspari AA. Rituximab for the treatment of recalcitrant chronic autoimmune urticaria. J Drugs Dermatol 2015;14:1387.
74. Mallipedi R, Grattan CE. Lack of response of severe steroid-dependent chronic urticaria to Rituximab. Clin Exp Dermatol 2007;32:333–4.
75. Ghazan-Shahi S, Ellis AK. Severe steroid-dependent idiopathic angioedema with response to Rituximab. Ann Allergy Asthma Immunol 2011;107:374–6.
76. Kocatürk E, Maurer M, Metz M, et al. Looking forward to new targeted treatments for chronic spontaneous urticaria. Clin Transl Allergy 2017;7:1.
77. Kiwamoto T, Kawasaki N, Paulson JS, et al. Siglec-8 as a drugable target to treat eosinophil and mast cell-associated conditions. Pharmacol Ther 2012;135: 327–36.
78. Altrichter S, Staubach P, Pasha M, et al. Clinical activity of AK002, an anti-Siglec-8 antibody, in multiple forms of uncontrolled chronic urticaria. Ann Allergy Asthma Immunol 2019;123:S27–8.
79. Kay AB, Clark P, Maurer M, et al. Elevations in T-helper-2-initiating cytokines (interleukin-33, interleukin-25 and thymic stromal lymphopoietin) in lesional skin from chronic spontaneous (idiopathic) urticaria. Br J Dermatol 2015;172: 1294–302.
80. Lee JK, Simpson RS. Dupilumab as a novel therapy for difficult to treat chronic spontaneous urticaria. J Allergy Clin Immunol Pract 2019;7:1659–61.
81. Kay AB, Ying S, Ardelean E, et al. Elevations in vascular markers and eosinophils in chronic spontaneous urticarial weals with low level persistence in uninvolved skin. Br J Dermatol 2014;171:505–11.
82. Tedeschi A, Kolkhir P, Asero R, et al. Chronic urticaria and coagulation: Pathophysiological and clinical aspects. Allergy 2014;69:683–91.
83. Magerl M, Terhorst D, Metz M, et al. Benefit of Mepolizumab treatment in a patient with chronic spontaneous urticaria. J Deutsch Dermatol Ges 2018;16:477–8.
84. Maurer M, Altrichter S, Metz M, et al. Benefit from Reslizumab treatment in a patient with chronic spontaneous urticaria and cold urticaria. J Eur Acad Dermatol Venereol 2018;32:e112–3.
85. Caproni M, Cardinali C, Giomi B, et al. Serological detection of eotaxin, IL-4, IL-13, interferon-gamma, MIP-1 alpha, TARC and IP-10 in chronic autoimmune urticaria and chronic idiopathic urticaria. J Dermatol Sci 2004;36:57–9.
86. Bae Y, Izuhara K, Ohta S, et al. Periostin and interleukin-13 are independently related to chronic spontaneous urticaria. Allergy Asthma Immunol Res 2016;8: 457–60.

Biologic Agents for the Treatment of Anaphylaxis

Luciana Kase Tanno, MD, PhD[a,b,c,d,*], Bryan Martin, DO[e,1]

KEYWORDS

• Anaphylaxis • Biologic agents • Biotherapy • Management • Treatment

KEY POINTS

• Adrenaline is still the initial treatment of choice in all cases of anaphylaxis and its administration should not be delayed.

• Developments in anaphylaxis have consistently followed pharmacologic developments offering possibilities of better management and prevention.

• Avoidance of trigger exposure and adrenaline administration remain the mainstay of long-term control of anaphylaxis; however, inadvertent exposure to allergens always remains a possibility.

• Biological agents as single medications or as combined therapy with food or venom immunotherapy, are effective as preventive treatments to reduce the most severe anaphylactic reactions.

• Cost-effectiveness of the use of biologic agents in anaphylaxis should be considered individually.

ANAPHYLAXIS: A HIGH-PRIORITY PUBLIC HEALTH ISSUE THAT REQUIRES IMMEDIATE TREATMENT AND PREVENTIVE MEASURES
Anaphylaxis: a High-Priority Public Health Issue

Since the term anaphylaxis was first coined in 1902 by Charles Richet and Paul Portier,[1] it has rapidly spread all around the world and its clinical importance as an emergency condition is now well accepted. Anaphylaxis is currently clinically defined as a

Conflicts of interest: The authors have no conflicts of interest related to the contents of this article.

Funding: L.K. Tanno received an unrestricted Novartis and MEDA/Mylan Pharma grants through CHRUM administration.

[a] Hospital Sírio-Libanês; [b] University Hospital of Montpellier, Montpellier, France; [c] Sorbonne Université, INSERM UMR-S 1136, IPLESP, Equipe EPAR, Paris 75013, France; [d] WHO Collaborating Centre on Scientific Classification Support, Montpellier, France; [e] Department of Medicine, The Ohio State University, 410 West 10th Avenue, Columbus, OH 43210, USA

[1] Present address: 2050 Kenny Road Suite 2200, Columbus, OH 43221.

* Corresponding author. Division of Allergy, Department of Pulmonology, Hôpital Arnaud de Villeneuve, University Hospital of Montpellier, 371, av. du Doyen Gaston Giraud, Montpellier Cedex 5 34295, France.

E-mail address: luciana.tanno@gmail.com

Immunol Allergy Clin N Am 40 (2020) 625–633
https://doi.org/10.1016/j.iac.2020.06.006
0889-8561/20/© 2020 Elsevier Inc. All rights reserved.

immunology.theclinics.com

severe, life-threatening systemic hypersensitivity reaction characterized by rapid onset and the potential to endanger life through airway, breathing, or circulatory problems[2–7] that require prompt identification and treatment.

Anaphylaxis is a syndrome with a constellation of features and signs that can manifest at any age, with multiple triggers, and any health professional may face it. Thus, patients with anaphylaxis have a chronic condition with intermittent and potentially fatal acute events. The treatment of anaphylaxis primarily comprises medications at the acute phase (mainly adrenaline) and then long-term avoidance and prevention measures.

The reported rate of occurrence seems to vary widely from one country to another. The lifetime prevalence has been estimated at 0.05% to 2% based on international studies.[8] In a recent systematic review of the global incidence and prevalence of anaphylaxis in children, the investigators reviewed 59 studies from 20 countries and the range of total anaphylaxis incidence ranged from 1 to 761 per 100,000 person years.[9] Anaphylaxis is a recognized cause of death in all ages, with the anaphylaxis-related mortality less than 1 per million per year in most high-income countries.[10–18] There are limited epidemiologic data from middle-income and low-income countries. Deaths from anaphylaxis are difficult to investigate because of misdiagnosis and miscoding, but morbidity and mortality statistics on anaphylaxis may gain new perspectives with the implementation of the eleventh version of the World Health Organization (WHO) International Classification of Diseases, in which anaphylaxis is now better represented.[19–22]

Because of varied, multidimensional clinical presentations, risk of fatality, and sudden onset in any setting, the allergy community has designated anaphylaxis as a high-priority public health issue.

From Clinical Anaphylaxis to Endotypes

The clinical definition, classification, nomenclature, and treatment of anaphylaxis have been points of controversy among different medical subspecialties and in different countries. Therefore, it became clear that an important goal would be to achieve a true international consensus. For this reason, multinational and multidisciplinary collaboration, led by allergy academies, resulted in the International Consensus on Anaphylaxis.[7]

From the initial description of anaphylaxis as a clinical entity with acute onset of symptoms involving 2 or more organs or association with hypotension or upper respiratory, its definition has evolved in recent publications to a more mechanistic description based on precision medicine classifying phenotypes with underlying endotypes supported by diagnostic biomarkers. At present, anaphylaxis phenotypes are defined by clinical presentation into type I–like reactions, cytokine storm–like reactions, and mixed reactions. The endotypes underlying these phenotypes include immunoglobulin (Ig) E–mediated and non–IgE-mediated mechanisms, cytokine release, mixed reactions, and direct activation of immune cells.[23,24] Better understanding of underlying mechanisms of anaphylaxis and the stratification of endotypes support precision medicine and may allow the integration of new therapeutic approaches, such as the use of biologic agents.

Anaphylaxis Treatment and Prevention: Current Status

In order to decrease the risk of death and optimize the treatment of anaphylaxis, all the guidelines[2–7] convey the need for a standardized protocol in which the removal of the trigger, the prompt initial pharmacologic treatment (epinephrine mainly), the appropriate positioning of the patient, and call for help should be started simultaneously.

Because anaphylaxis mimics common conditions, such as asthma and urticaria, and because it can present without hypotension, its diagnosis is often missed or delayed. As a consequence, this may lead to the delay of appropriate treatment, increasing the risk of death.

Adrenaline (epinephrine) is still the first-line treatment of any type of anaphylaxis and is recognized as the only medication documented to prevent hospitalizations, hypoxic sequelae, and fatalities. Glucocorticoids and antihistamines should be used only as third-line treatment in anaphylaxis treatment. Their administration should never delay adrenaline injection in anaphylaxis.[2–7,24,25] Delay in the use of adrenaline (recognized as a factor that may increase the risk of death in anaphylaxis) and the global availability of adrenaline autoinjectors are still key issues in the management of anaphylaxis.[26]

Because public health's core mission is prevention of injury or disease, there are many potential strategic interventions. Tertiary prevention strategies are the most familiar for physicians worldwide who are involved in clinical medicine. When applied to anaphylaxis, it is intended to reduce the risk of another reaction and/or manage it appropriately to avoid negative outcomes. Prevention of anaphylaxis depends primarily on optimal management of patient-related risk factors; strict avoidance of confirmed relevant allergens or triggers; and, where indicated, immunomodulation (eg, Hymenoptera venom immunotherapy). The use of biologic agents in anaphylaxis has been gaining interest over the last years.[25]

This article reviews the use of biologic agents used in the treatment of anaphylaxis with the view that new knowledge can support high-quality practice and empower allergists and health professionals with new tools that can be used to treat symptoms and prevent anaphylaxis.

IS THERE A PLACE FOR BIOLOGIC AGENTS IN ANAPHYLAXIS TREATMENT?
Monoclonal Agents: Current Status

The recent description of phenotypes provides new insight and understanding into the mechanisms and causes of anaphylaxis through a better understanding of endotypes and application of precision medicine. Several biologic therapies are emerging as potential preventive or adjuvant treatment of anaphylaxis.

The commercial use of monoclonal antibodies (mAbs) began in early 1980s, and the first therapeutic mAb targeting the immune system was approved in 1986.[27] In 2014, 47 mAbs were approved in the United States or Europe for the treatment of a variety of diseases, and many of these products have also been approved for the global market. It was estimated that there would be an approval rate of 4 new products per year and the availability of ~70 mAbs on the market by 2020, with worldwide sales of nearly $125 billion. At present, 200 biologic agents are commercially available for all conditions. These therapies are responsible for about 30% of all drugs under development.[27–31]

Overall Evidence Base for Anaphylaxis Treatment with Biologic Agents

Most biologic agents target respiratory conditions, but new drugs have emerged to cover other allergic and hypersensitivity conditions such as atopic dermatitis, and eosinophilic conditions such as eosinophilic esophagitis. Although biologic agents are still not licensed for the treatment of anaphylaxis, in recent years these drugs, in particular omalizumab (anti-IgE mAb), have been used as therapeutic adjuvants as a preventive treatment of anaphylaxis. At present, there are 63 clinical trials registered for anaphylaxis; only 3 involve omalizumab.[32]

Omalizumab is 95% humanized mAb that recognizes and binds to the Fc portion of the IgE molecule in order to block IgE binding to mast cells and basophils. It prevents IgE expression on allergic effector cells and subsequent allergen-induced cross-linking of IgE.[32] This treatment is now formally indicated for moderate to severe persistent allergic asthma with proven sensitization to perennial aeroallergen in patients refractory to usual treatment and for chronic idiopathic urticaria in patients who remain symptomatic despite H1 antihistamine treatment. Therapeutic strategies based on omalizumab administration in other disorders are currently only based on limited clinical trials, observations, case series, and expert opinions.[33]

Besides the formal indication of omalizumab for allergic asthma, this drug has also been shown to reduce the frequency and intensity of side effects when combined with allergen immunotherapy (AIT) to allergic rhinitis induced by grass pollen. A multicenter study showed that patients who received omalizumab had lower frequency of adverse events than the group receiving AIT alone. Post hoc analysis showed that the association of omalizumab resulted in a 5-fold decrease in the risk of AIT-induced anaphylaxis.[34]

mAbs can also induce hypersensitivity conditions, ranging from mild cutaneous reactions to life-threatening presentations. Recent data have provided evidence of successful desensitization to an increased number of mAbs, including rituximab, ofatumumab, obinutuzumab, trastuzumab, cetuximab, tocilizumab, infliximab, etanercept, adalimumab, golimumab, certolizumab, brentuximab, bevacizumab, and omalizumab.[24] However, mAbs can also be used as adjuvants in the desensitization to other drugs in order to reduce the severity of side effects during these procedures. Desensitization to antibiotics in combination with omalizumab has been successfully done in targeted populations, such as patients with cystic fibrosis, with a similar protocol as for chemotherapy drugs. Desensitization to aspirin combined with omalizumab for aspirin-exacerbated respiratory disease has provided increased sense of smell, prevented the regrowth of polyps, and helped stabilize asthma symptoms.

Omalizumab is a potential adjuvant in food oral immunotherapy. A recent phase 2 randomized, double-blind, placebo-controlled trial of 37 peanut-allergic children undergoing oral immunotherapy showed that omalizumab administration (12 weeks) allowed tolerance of 2000 mg of peanut on discontinuation of immunotherapy more often than placebo (74% vs 13%, $P<.01$).[35] Participants assigned to omalizumab were also less likely to experience adverse reactions to peanut immunotherapy. Omalizumab, administered solely or in combination for 28 months, was also shown to improve safety but not efficacy in 57 subjects (7–32 years old) with a cow's milk allergy undergoing oral immunotherapy.[36] A phase 1 randomized trial performed with children with proven multiple food allergies suggested that omalizumab in combination with oral immunotherapy with multiple food allergens was able to reduce the time to reach the target dose and to minimize the severe symptoms during the procedure.[37]

Omalizumab has been shown to be a successful treatment of idiopathic anaphylaxis, effectively reducing the number of episodes and improving the quality of life.[38–41] Patients with idiopathic anaphylaxis who were not controlled despite continuous use of oral corticosteroids and/or antihistamines were treated with omalizumab (300–375 mg every 2–4 weeks) for 10 to 14 months.[38–41] In these 4 patients, no anaphylaxis episode was recorded after onset of omalizumab injection. Omalizumab may be a preventive therapeutic option in patients with idiopathic anaphylaxis depending on the severity and frequency of episodes, but the cost/benefit ratio should be assessed individually.

Mastocytosis and mast cell activation disorders may be identified as a cause of idiopathic anaphylaxis.[40] Omalizumab has been shown also to reduce anaphylaxis episodes and skin symptoms and increase quality of life in 13 adult patients with systemic mastocytosis who received this treatment with a median duration of 17 months (range, 1–73 months).[42,43]

Hymenoptera venom immunotherapy is indicated in patients with sting anaphylaxis. Patients with mast cell activation disorders or mastocytosis who developed sting anaphylaxis can also receive venom immunotherapy. However, in these patients, the venom immunotherapy is likely to provide incomplete protection and the patient may have increased adverse reactions. Pretreatment with omalizumab has been shown to be effective as an adjunctive treatment in patients with mastocytosis, used for both symptom improvement and to dampen adverse effects caused by venom immunotherapy.[44–51]

New Monoclonal Antibodies, New Perspectives?

Although anaphylaxis is not only IgE mediated, new mAbs targeting IgE are being studied and may be possible adjuvants in the management and prevention of anaphylaxis in the future.

Ligelizumab is a humanized IgG1 mAb that binds to the Ce3 domain of IgE193.[52] A recent phase 2b study evaluated the efficacy and safety of this drug in patients with moderate/severe urticaria, with positive outcomes.[53] Phase 3 studies are ongoing, but there is still no study involving anaphylactic patients.[54]

Quilizumab is a humanized mAb that targets the main segment M1 (M1 prime segment) of IgE expressed on the membrane of B cells and plasmablasts with an IgE switch.[54] In clinical studies in healthy volunteers and patients with asthma and rhinitis, quilizumab reduced the levels of total and specific IgE and sustained them for at least 6 weeks.[55] In a small study with patients with refractory urticaria, quilizumab showed no significant benefits in changing the pruritus score. The investigators speculate that higher doses or longer treatment could have provided a more efficient response.[56] Although targeting IgE expression, there are still no registered studies in anaphylaxis.

BIOLOGIC AGENTS AND ANAPHYLAXIS

The recent description of phenotypes provides new insight and understanding into the mechanisms and causes of anaphylaxis through a better understanding of endotypes and application of precision medicine. Several biologic therapies and new devices are emerging as potential preventive treatment of anaphylaxis. However, adrenaline (epinephrine) is still the first-line treatment of any type of anaphylaxis.

Biologic drugs, such as omalizumab, have been used as therapeutic adjuvants as a preventive treatment of anaphylaxis, but cost-effectiveness should be considered individually. Real-world questions about safety and effectiveness of such novel approaches remain unclear. The cost of such medications and knowledge gaps about long-term benefit/risk, adherence, and comparative effectiveness require further research and expertise.

CLINICS CARE POINTS

- Acute anaphylaxis is often underdiagnosed and undertreated.
- Adrenaline (epinephrine) is the treatment of choice for anaphylaxis; therapy should begin at 0.01 mg/kg up to a dose of 0.5 mg.
- Glucocorticoids and antihistamines are not part of the initial treatment of acute anaphylaxis. Epinephrine administration should not be delayed in order to initiate therapy with these agents.

- After treatment of the acute event, anaphylaxis should be treated as a chronic condition with the potential for life-threatening exacerbations. Although avoidance is the mainstay for long-term control of anaphylaxis, inadvertent exposure to allergens is always a possibility.
- Understanding the underlying endotypes of anaphylaxis may lead to new therapeutic options.

REFERENCES

1. Portier P, Richet C. De l'action anaphylactique de certains venins. C R Seances Soc Biol 1902;54:170.
2. Sampson HA, Munoz-Furlong A, Campbell RL, et al. Second symposium on the definition and management of anaphylaxis: summary report – Second National Institute of Allergy and Infectious Disease/Food Allergy and Anaphylaxis Network Symposium. J Allergy Clin Immunol 2006;117:391–7.
3. Muraro A, Roberts G, Worm M, et al. Anaphylaxis: guidelines from the European Academy of Allergy and Clinical Immunology. Allergy 2014;69:1026–45.
4. Lieberman P, Nicklas RA, Oppenheimer J, et al. The diagnosis and management of anaphylaxis practice parameter: 2010 update. J Allergy Clin Immunol 2010; 126:477–80.
5. Simons FER, Ardusso LRF, Bilò MB, et al. World Allergy Organization guidelines for the assessment and management of anaphylaxis. World Allergy Organ J 2011;4:13–37.
6. Brown SG, Mullins RJ, Gold MS. Anaphylaxis: diagnosis and management. Med J Aust 2006;185:283–9.
7. Simons FER, Ardusso LR, Bilò MB, et al. International consensus on (ICON) Anaphylaxis. World Allergy Organ J 2014;30(7):9.
8. Wang Y, Allen KJ, Suaini NHA, et al. The global incidence and prevalence of anaphylaxis in children in the general population: A systematic review. Allergy 2019;74:1063–80.
9. Panesar SS, Javad S, de Silva D, et al. A on behalf of the EAACI Food Allergy and Anaphylaxis Group. The epidemiology of anaphylaxis in Europe: a systematic review. Allergy 2013;68:1353–61.
10. Turner PJ, Gowland MH, Sharma V, et al. Increase in anaphylaxis-related hospitalizations but no increase in fatalities: an analysis of United Kingdom national anaphylaxis data, 1992-2012. J Allergy Clin Immunol 2015;135:956–63.
11. Ma L, Danoff TM, Borish L. Case fatality and population mortality associated with anaphylaxis in the United States. J Allergy Clin Immunol 2014;133:1075–83.
12. Lin RY, Anderson AS, Shah SN, et al. Increasing anaphylaxis hospitalizations in the first 2 decades of life: New York State, 1990-2006. Ann Allergy Asthma Immunol 2008;101:387–93.
13. Brown AF, McKinnon D, Chu K. Emergency department anaphylaxis: A review of 142 patients in a single year. J Allergy Clin Immunol 2001;108:861–6.
14. Poulos LM, Waters AM, Correll PK, et al. Trends in hospitalizations for anaphylaxis, angioedema, and urticaria in Australia, 1993-1994 to 2004-2005. J Allergy Clin Immunol 2007;120:878–84.
15. Mullins RJ, Wainstein BK, Barnes EH, et al. Increases in anaphylaxis fatalities in Australia from 1997 to 2013. Clin Exp Allergy 2016;46:1099–110.
16. Jerschow E, Lin RY, Scaperotti MM, et al. Fatal anaphylaxis in the United States, 1999-2010: temporal patterns and demographic associations. J Allergy Clin Immunol 2014;134:1318–28.

17. Pouessel G, Claverie C, Labreuche J, et al. Fatal anaphylaxis in France: Analysis of national anaphylaxis data, 1979-2011. J Allergy Clin Immunol 2017. https://doi.org/10.1016/j.jaci.2017.02.014.

18. Tanno LK, Ganem F, Demoly P, et al. Undernotification of anaphylaxis deaths in Brazil due to difficult coding under the ICD-10. Allergy 2012;67:783–9.

19. Tanno LK, Bierrenbach AL, Calderon MA, et al. Joint Allergy Academies. Decreasing the undernotification of anaphylaxis deaths in Brazil through the International Classification of Diseases (ICD)-11 revision. Allergy 2017;72:120–5.

20. Tanno LK, Calderon MA, Demoly P, on behalf the Joint Allergy Academies. New Allergic and Hypersensitivity Conditions Section in the International Classification of Diseases-11. Allergy Asthma Immunol Res 2016;8(4):383–8.

21. Tanno LK, Molinari N, Bruel S, et al. Joint Allergy Academies. Field-testing the New Anaphylaxis' Classification for the WHO International Classification of Diseases (ICD)-11 Revision. Allergy 2017;72(5):820–6.

22. Tanno LK, Chalmers R, Bierrenbach AL, et al, on behalf Joint Allergy Academies. Changing the history of anaphylaxis mortality statistics through the World Health Organization's International Classification of Diseases (ICD)-11. J Allergy Clin Immunol 2019;144(3):627–33.

23. Castells M. Diagnosis and management of anaphylaxis in precision medicine. J Allergy Clin Immunol 2017;140(2):321–33.

24. Jimenez-Rodriguez TW, Garcia-Neuer M, Alenazy LA, et al. Anaphylaxis in the 21st century: phenotypes, endotypes, and biomarkers. J Asthma Allergy 2018; 11:121–42.

25. Tanno LK, Alvarez-Perea A, Pouessel G. Therapeutic approach in anaphylaxis. Curr Opin Allergy Clin Immunol 2019;19(4):393–401.

26. Tanno LK, Simons FER, Sanchez-Borges M, et al. Joint Allergy Academies. Applying prevention concepts to anaphylaxis: A call for worldwide availability of adrenaline auto-injectors. Clin Exp Allergy 2017;47(9):1108–14.

27. Ecker DM, Jones SD, Levine HL. The therapeutic monoclonal antibody market. MAbs 2015;7(1):9–14.

28. Bioprocess Technology Consultants website Woburn (MA): Bioprocess Technology Consultants, Inc. bioTRAK® database. 2014. Available at: http://www.bptc.com/pipeline-databases.php.

29. Pharmaceutical Research and Manufacturers of America. Medicines in development: biologics 2013 report. Washington, DC: Pharmaceutical Research and Manufacturers of America; 2013. Available at: http://www.phrma.org/sites/default/files/pdf/biologics2013.pdf.

30. Drugs@FDA [Internet] Silver Spring (MD): U.S. Food and Drug Administration, Center for Drug Evaluation and Research. Available at: http://www.accessdata.fda.gov/scripts/cder/drugsatfda/index.cfm.

31. European public assessment reports, human medicines. London: The European Medicines Agency. 1995. Available at: http://www.ema.europa.eu/ema/index.jsp?curl=pages/medicines/landing/epar_search.jsp&mid=WC0b01ac058001d124.

32. Casale TB, Stokes JR. Immunomodulators for allergic respiratory disorders. J Allergy Clin Immunol 2008;121:288–96.

33. Cardet JC, Casale TB. New Insights into the Utility of Omalizumab. J Allergy Clin Immunol 2019. https://doi.org/10.1016/j.jaci.2019.01.016 [pii:S0091–6749(19)30111-3].

34. Casale TB, Busse WW, Kline JN, et al. Omalizumab pretreatment decreases acute reactions after rush immunotherapy for ragweed-induced seasonal allergic rhinitis. J Allergy Clin Immunol 2006;117:134–40.

35. MacGinnitle AJ, Rachid R, Gragg H, et al. Omalizumab facilitates rapid oral desensitization for peanut allergy. J Allergy Clin Immunol 2017;139:873–81.e8.
36. Wood RA. Advances in food allergy in 2015. J Allergy Clin Immunol 2016;138: 1541–7.
37. Bégin P, Dominguez T, Wilson SP, et al. Phase 1 results of safety and tolerability in a rush oral immunotherapy protocol to multiple foods using Omalizumab. Allergy Asthma Clin Immunol 2014;10:7.
38. Pitt TJ, Cisneros N, Kalicinsky C, et al. Successful treatment of idiopathic anaphylaxis in an adolescent. J Allergy Clin Immunol 2010;126:415–6.
39. Warrier P, Casale TB. Omalizumab in idiopathic anaphylaxis. Ann Allergy Asthma Immunol 2009;102:257–8.
40. Jones JD, Marney SR Jr, Fahrenholz JM. Idiopathic anaphylaxis successfully treated with omalizumab. Ann Allergy Asthma Immunol 2008;101:550–1.
41. Demirtürk M, Gelincik A, Colakoğlu B, et al. Promising option in the prevention of idiopathic anaphylaxis: omalizumab. J Dermatol 2012;39:552–4.
42. Lieberman PL, Umetsu DT, Carrigan GJ, et al. Anaphylactic reactions associated with omalizumab administration: Analysis of a case-control study. J Allergy Clin Immunol 2016;138:913–5.e2.
43. Broesby-Olsen S, Vestergaard H, Mortz CG, et al, Mastocytosis Centre Odense University Hospital (MastOUH). Omalizumab prevents anaphylaxis and improves symptoms in systemic mastocytosis: Efficacy and safety observations. Allergy 2018;73:230–8.
44. Palgan K, Bartuzi Z, Gotz-Zbikowska M. Treatment with a combination of omalizumab and specific immunotherapy for severe anaphylaxis after a wasp sting. Int J Immunopathol Pharmacol 2014;27:109–12.
45. da Silva EN, Randall KL. Omalizumab mitigates anaphylaxis during ultrarush honey bee venom immunotherapy in monoclonal mast cell activation syndrome. J Allergy Clin Immunol Pract 2013;1:687–8.
46. Slaughter EM, Boyer N, Bennett S. The bee sting that was not: an unusual case of hymenoptera anaphylaxis averted in a patient treated with omalizumab for asthma. Case Rep Med 2014;2014:138963.
47. Galera C, Soohun N, Zankar N, et al. Severe anaphylaxis to bee venom immunotherapy: efficacy of pretreatment and concurrent treatment with omalizumab. J Investig Allergol Clin Immunol 2009;19:225–9.
48. Castells MC, Hornick JL, Akin C. Anaphylaxis after hymenoptera sting: is it venom allergy, a clonal disorder, or both? J Allergy Clin Immunol Pract 2015;3:350–5.
49. Sokol KC, Ghazi A, Kelly BC, et al. Omalizumab as a desensitizing agent and treatment in mastocytosis: a review of the literature and case report. J Allergy Clin Immunol Pract 2014;2:266–70.
50. Carter MC, Robyn JA, Bressler PB, et al. Omalizumab for the treatment of unprovoked anaphylaxis in patients with systemic mastocytosis. J Allergy Clin Immunol 2007;119:1550–1.
51. Ricciardi L. Omalizumab: a useful tool for inducing tolerance to bee venom immunotherapy. Int J Immunopathol Pharmacol 2016;29:726–8.
52. Arm JP, Bottoli I, Skerjanec A, et al. Pharmacokinetics, pharmacodynamics and safety of QGE031 (ligelizumab), a novel high-affinity anti-IgE antibody, in atopic subjects. Clin Exp Allergy 2014;44(11):1371–85.
53. Maurer M, Gimenez-Arnau A, Sussman G, et al. Ligelizumab as add on therapy for patients with H1 antihistamine refractory chronic spontaneous urticaria: Primary results of a placebo and active controlled phase 2b dose finding study. Allergy 2018;73(S105):837.

54. ClinicalTrials. gov website. Bethesda (MD): National Library of Medicine (US). Available.   Available   at: https://clinicaltrials.gov/ct2/results?cond=&term= ligelizumab&cntry=&state=&city=&dist=. Accessed January, 2020.
55. Harris JM, Maciuca R, Bradley MS, et al. A randomized trial of the efficacy and safety of quilizumab in adults with inadequately controlled allergic asthma. Respir Res 2016;17:29.
56. Harris JM, Cabanski CR, Scheerens H, et al. A randomized trial of quilizumab in adults with refractory chronic spontaneous urticaria. J Allergy Clin Immunol 2016; 138:1730–2.

Immune-Related Adverse Drug Reactions and Immunologically Mediated Drug Hypersensitivity

Eric Macy, MD, MS*

KEYWORDS

- Adverse drug reaction • Adenovirus vector • Allergy • Complement
- Cytokine storm • Gene transfer • Hypersensitivity • Hypogammaglobulinemia

KEY POINTS

- Therapeutic agents used to treat immunologically mediated conditions can cause immunologically mediated adverse reactions because the immune system may recognize the therapeutic agent as not-self or because the therapeutic agent can have a disruptive effect on normal immune system function.
- The time to onset of the adverse reaction and the clinical characteristics of the reaction are the key features that help determine the mechanism of the adverse reaction, guide appropriate testing to confirm the mechanism, and then direct subsequent management.
- Reexposure to therapeutic agents used to treat immunologically mediated conditions that have been associated with an adverse reaction may be appropriate if there is no useful alternative for a potentially life-threatening condition, the patient is willing to experience another reaction of similar severity to the index reaction, and the treating physicians are able to manage subsequent reactions.
- Desensitization is only reliably useful in the setting of immunoglobulin E–mediated acute-onset hypersensitivity. It may be possible to treat through mild T-cell–mediated reactions, but it is currently not possible to desensitize these individuals.

INTRODUCTION

This review concentrates on the essential practical elements currently needed to understand and manage immune-related adverse drug reactions and immunologically mediated drug hypersensitivity, with an emphasis on biologics used for the treatment of immune-mediated hypersensitivity conditions. This includes how to proceed when a suspected immune-related adverse drug reaction and immunologically mediated

Southern California Permanente Medical Group, Kaiser Permanente Southern California, San Diego Medical Center, San Diego, CA, USA
* Allergy Department, 7060 Clairemont Mesa Boulevard, San Diego, CA 92111.
E-mail address: eric.m.macy@kp.org
Twitter: @EricMacyMD (E.M.)

Immunol Allergy Clin N Am 40 (2020) 635–647
https://doi.org/10.1016/j.iac.2020.06.003
0889-8561/20/© 2020 Elsevier Inc. All rights reserved.
immunology.theclinics.com

drug hypersensitivity is already noted in the medical record, how to treat immune-related adverse drug reactions or immunologically mediated drug hypersensitivity during therapy, and how to potentially prevent immune-related adverse drug reactions and immunologically mediated drug hypersensitivity from occurring when using biologicals or other therapeutic or diagnostic agents.

DEFINITIONS

The general term that best describes an inability to safely administer or re-administer a specific drug because of fear, preference, genetic, clinical, or metabolic considerations, or a previous adverse reaction associated with, attributed to, or caused by specific drug is intolerance.[1] Most reported drug intolerances, commonly mislabeled as an "allergy" in the electronic health record (EHR) are just expected side effects.[2] It is important not to expose susceptible individuals to specific drugs when a contraindicating physiologic or genetic condition is present, such as certain HLA haplotypes, enzyme abnormalities, or co-usage of another medication that effects enzyme function or metabolism. Only a small fraction of what are typically reported in the EHR as drug "allergy" have anything to do with the immune system.[3] Only a subgroup of these are because of antigen-specific hypersensitivity, and only a very small group are from clinically significant immunoglobulin (Ig)E-mediated allergy.[4] It is also possible to have immune-related adverse drug reactions from medications interacting with immune system cells or proteins through antigen nonspecific mechanisms resulting in generalized pathologic immune activation or suppression.

Immunologically mediated drug hypersensitivity refers to the limited subset of adverse drug reactions that are mediated through antigen-specific immunoglobulins or antigen-specific T lymphocytes.[5] Antigen-specific immunoglobulins, including IgG, which may or may not be able to activate the complement system, and IgE, which when bound to mast cells can be cross-linked by polyvalent antigen exposure and induce urticaria or anaphylaxis through acute mast cell activation and mediator release. Antigen-specific T cells can be activated by peptide fragments via the T-cell antigen receptor (TCR), which is composed of a ligand-binding subunit, the α and β chains, and a signaling subunit, namely the $CD3\varepsilon$, γ, and δ chains and the $TCR\zeta$ chain.[6] T cells can also be activated by the noncovalent pharmacologic interaction of small molecules with distinct HLA molecules or TCRs, the p-i concept.[7] P-i reactions differ from other off-target adverse drug reactions, as the reaction is not due to the effect on the drug-modified cells themselves, but is the consequence of reactive T cells.

The word "allergy" needs to be reserved to describe clinically significant antigen-specific IgE-mediated acute-onset hypersensitivity that can be desensitized.[1,5] A person with a positive skin test result or serum IgE test result does not have a drug allergy unless the person also experiences clinically significant acute-onset hives or more serious IgE-mediated systemic symptoms, such as hypotension or shortness of breath: anaphylaxis, with a full-dose reexposure. If a person has acute-onset mild hives, or even a benign maculopapular rash, associated with oral exposure to an antibiotic and needs that specific antibiotic for a several-day course, it is often OK to continue the course uninterrupted and treat through the benign reaction.[5] This is functionally the same as having hives during a desensitization and continuing to treat through to a therapeutic dose. It is critical not to stop a medication suspected of inducing IgE, wait more than 5 half-lives, and then restart the same medication at a therapeutic dose, because of an elevated risk of inducing anaphylaxis. With most small molecules that need to haptenate serum proteins to trigger immune reactions, anaphylaxis is extremely rare. With intact antigens, such as therapeutic proteins, such as biologicals, anaphylaxis is much more common. Anaphylaxis is still often over-coded in EHRs.[8] When evaluating the incidence of medication-associated anaphylaxis through EHR coding, it is essential to audit the actual event, and not just tabulate the codes.

Using the word "allergy" to describe delayed-onset T-cell–mediated hypersensitivity may result in therapeutic mis-adventures, such as performing puncture or intradermal skin testing and reading the results 15 minute later or even worse, attempting a desensitization.[5] It may be possible to treat through mild T-cell–mediated reactions, but it is not possible to alter clinically significant T-cell–mediated reactions by administering doubling doses of a medication, unlike mast cell–mediated reactions triggered by antigen-specific IgE. Serious cutaneous and systemic adverse drug reactions (SCARs) are fortunately extremely rare, even with biologicals. Stevens-Johnson syndrome (SJS) is often overdiagnosed.[9] Suspected SCARs should always be biopsied, and laboratory testing for eosinophilia and liver enzymes should be obtained.[2]

The elements of the immune system, including cells and serum proteins, function as biologic amplifiers. They can act through antigen-specific reactions, antibody and T-cell receptors, and also through direct effects of drugs interacting with a variety of surface and intracellular receptors on lymphocytes, mast cells, basophils, eosinophils, neutrophils, and platelets, and the proteins that make up the classic and alternative complement pathways.

Pichler[10] in 2006 reviewed adverse side effects associated with the use of protein biological agents. He grouped these adverse side effects into 5 groups: type α, cytokine release syndrome; type β, immune-mediated reactions against the agent; type γ, immune or cytokine imbalance; type δ, cross-reactivity; and type ε, non–immunologically associated side effects.[10] Please see **Table 1**.

BACKGROUND

Most of what is labeled as drug allergy in the medical record, when referring to nonprotein small molecules, has nothing to do with IgE-mediated allergy or even

Table 1
Pichler's grouping of adverse side-effects of biologic agents

	Categories	Mechanisms
Type α	Cytokine release syndrome Cytokine storm	a. Capillary leak b. Endothelial damage c. Disseminated intravascular coagulation
Type β	Immune-mediated	a. Immunoglobulin (Ig)E-mediated allergy b. T-cell–mediated hypersensitivity
Type γ	Immune or cytotoxic imbalance	a. Impaired immune function, immunodeficiency, resulting in infections b. Autoimmunity c. Induce IgE-mediated allergy to another antigen
Type δ	Cross-reactivity	Exogenously produced antitumor monoclonal antibodies binding to antigens on normal cells causing their death or dysfunction
Type ε	Nonimmunologic side effects	Binding to the intended target of the biologic agent in nontargeted cells, such as in nervous system, endocrine tissue, or the heart, resulting in unintended side effects

Data from Pichler WJ. Adverse side-effects to biological agents. Allergy 2006;61:912-20.

immunologically mediated drug hypersensitivity. IgE-mediated immune responses are primarily possible against small molecules that are able to covalently bind to serum proteins. The classic examples are penicillins and other beta-lactams that are able to bind to serine, their target in bacterial penicillin binding proteins, and also present on human serum albumin and on other serum proteins. Molecules that are not covalently serum protein bound, such as macrolide antibiotics, are very much less likely to induce IgE-mediated allergy. The rate of immunologically mediated adverse reactions can vary widely with the same drug depending on how it is stored and the route of administration. A classic example are the penicillins, which are unstable in aqueous phase.[11] Aged penicillins in aqueous solutions administered parenterally induce much higher rates of antibody-mediated hypersensitivity than the same molecules administered as a pill orally. Many biological therapeutics used to treat immune-mediated hypersensitivity conditions are proteins capable of directly triggering the production of antigen-specific immunoglobulins, including IgE.

The key elements of an IgE-mediated drug allergy are as follows.[5] Previous exposure is needed to sensitize. Although cross-reactivity is often considered or hypothesized as possible, it is rarely confirmed. The reaction typically starts to occur within minutes of the first dose of the exposure.[12] Shorter times to the start of the reaction are noted after parenteral exposures compared with oral exposures. The reactions can vary from benign hives to life-threatening anaphylaxis. There is a threshold dose needed to trigger a reaction, and this may be as low as 1/2000th of a typical therapeutic dose. Individuals with confirmed IgE-mediated drug allergy who need the drug can be desensitized by administration of doubling doses, starting at approximately 1/2000th of the needed therapeutic dose.[5] True IgE-mediated hypersensitivity can wane with time. A positive skin test or in vitro–specific IgE antibody test result does not define a clinically significant allergy, one must also have clinically significant IgE-mediated symptoms, hives or anaphylaxis, with reexposure. False positive skin test results are common, and more common the smaller the wheal size used to define a positive test result. In general, at least 5 to 7 mm of wheal with flare greater than wheal is the minimum threshold that should be used to diagnose a clinically significant IgE-mediated drug allergy when skin testing, using a reagent concentration that does not induce this size of a wheal in a large group of individuals who tolerate the medication.

Timing is everything in the history. Blumenthal has noted that 2 significant risk factors for a confirmed IgE-mediated allergy are a history of anaphylaxis as the index event and onset of symptoms in less than 1 hour.[12] The key question in evaluating a reported drug intolerance is how long after the first dose of the last course did the adverse reaction start to appear. The international consensus for immediate-onset hypersensitivity is less than 6 hours, but with parenteral medications it is almost always within 30 minutes, and with oral medications causing clinically significant IgE-mediated allergy, within 1 hour.[2]

HISTORY

There are 2 highly feared immunologically mediated adverse reactions: IgE-mediated anaphylaxis and T-cell–mediated serious systemic reactions or SCARs.[5,13]

Anaphylaxis is defined as a multisystem affected syndrome caused by mast cell degranulation. It can be caused by an IgE-mediated mechanism, but also by direct mast cell activation without any IgE involvement. The alternative mechanisms include antigen-specific IgG activating complement, specifically C5a, and direct binding of a small molecule, such as a fluroquinolone antibiotic, to mast cell receptors, most significantly MRGPRX2, or via the cyclooxygenase (COX) pathway, as is seen with nonsteroidal anti-inflammatory drug (NSAID) hypersensitivity.[14,15]

SCARs include drug eruption and systemic symptoms (DRESS), SJS, and toxic epidermal necrolysis (TEN). SJS can also occur after infections, independent of any specific drug administration. SJS and even SJS/TEN overlap is often overdiagnosed or misdiagnosed. It is essential to obtain a skin biopsy, liver enzyme measurements, and a peripheral blood eosinophil count when DRESS/SJS/TEN is suspected to confirm the correct diagnosis.[13] With SJS/TEN it is also important to carefully quantitate the percentage of body surface area affected to determine the mortality risk. TEN is defined as at least 30% body surface area skin loss, typically requires management in a burn unit, and has a high death rate, often greater than 30%. SJS syndrome can be managed with careful nursing care in a general medical unit, as noted by work done in South Africa in patients positive for human immunodeficiency virus who required rechallenges with anti-tuberculosis (TB) drugs for multiple drug-resistant TB.[13] SCARs are more common in children with complex chronic conditions, and up to 16.7% of children hospitalized with SJS or TEN have at least 1 currently active underlying chronic complex conditions. The most commonly associated chronic complex conditions are metabolic, cardiac, or neurologic. The least commonly associated chronic complex conditions are malignancy, respiratory, or renal.

With DRESS syndrome it is important to be aware that severe systemic delayed-onset life-threatening eosinophilic inflammation of the heart is possible, even without any further drug exposure. Bourgeois and coworkers[16] in 2010 reviewed DRESS-associated myocarditis and noted that it can occur with initial DRESS symptoms onset or with a delay of up to 4 months. The severe version, acute necrotizing eosinophilic myocarditis, has a mortality rate of up to 50% and medial survival of only 3 to 4 days. Ventricular assist devices can be life-saving and allow cardiac recovery while the eosinophilic inflammation is treated.

Immune-related adverse events (irAEs) associated with the use of immune checkpoint inhibitors (ICIs), programmed death inhibitors (PDLs), and cytotoxic T-cell–associated protein-4 inhibitors are being increasing recognized.[17] The primary systemic targets are liver, endocrine, and renal.[18] Autoantibody production can also occur. Women typically report more immune-related adverse events. Chronic inflammatory arthritis can occur in 3% to 6% of people treated with ICIs.[19] Combining tumor necrosis factor (TNF) or interleukin (IL)-6 inhibitors with ICIs may both increase the effectiveness of the ICI therapy and reduce irAEs.[19]

EPIDEMIOLOGY

Female individuals report more drug intolerances than male individuals.[20] Drug "allergy" is baggage that accumulates with increasing age and higher levels of drug exposures. Drug "allergy" prevalence is particularly high in individuals with cystic fibrosis and cancer.[8] Individuals who have reported any drug "allergy" will report higher rates of new drug "allergy" with all drug exposures. Multiple drug intolerance syndrome, defined as ≥3 unrelated drug "allergy" reports is more common in female individuals and with increasing age.[20] Such individuals are not at any increased risk to be confirmed to have any specific drug-associated immunologically mediated hypersensitivity compared with individuals with only 1 specific reported drug intolerance. Even though women are more likely to report a penicillin "allergy," they are no more likely than men to be confirmed on testing.[21]

The rate of "allergy" reported to protein biological therapeutic agents is fairly high, often greater than 5%, compared with the rates of new "allergy" reported after NSAID, opiate, or antihypertension medication usage, typically less than 2% per course.[20] With most antibiotics, a new "allergy" is reported after approximately 0.5% to 4% of all exposures. Sulfonamide antibiotics routinely have the highest "allergy" rates and macrolide and tetracycline antibiotics are typically the lowest. Only a small fraction, typically approximately 10% for sulfonamides and approximately 3% for penicillins will be confirmed by rechallenge to have clinically significant immune-mediated hypersensitivity.[21,22] Individuals with a penicillin "allergy" who are subsequently delabeled after tolerating an oral challenge with a therapeutic dose are still approximately 2 to 3 times more likely to report a new "allergy" with each future therapeutic course compared with random patients with no reported drug intolerances.[23] But again, typically fewer than 3% will be confirmed to have developed a new immunologically mediated hypersensitivity if reevaluated.[24]

With angiotensin-converting enzyme inhibitors, the nonimmunologically mediated side effects of coughing and angioedema steadily increase with increased duration of use.[25]

With opiates, the rates of "allergy" reported are typically reflections of patient preference and the common side effect of direct mast cell activation and itching can be controlled by the co-use of nonsedating antihistamines. Constipation, respiratory depression, and central nervous system side effects are expected with all opiate use and are not necessarily contraindication to reuse.[20]

With adenovirus vectors used for gene transfer, the rate of humoral and cell-mediated immune reactions approach 100% with reexposure. These materials essentially function as adenovirus vaccines.[26]

MAST CELL ACTIVATION

There are multiple surface receptors on mast cells that can induce activation and mediator release including toll-like receptors, protease-activated receptors, and Mas-related G-protein coupled receptor member X2 (MRGPRX2).[14,27] Cofactors, such as temperature changes, NSAIDs, exercise, sleep deprivation, beta-blockers, angiotensin-converting enzyme inhibitors, and iodinated contrast media can exacerbate clinical symptoms and worsen anaphylaxis, independent of the triggering event.[28]

Direct mast cell activation through the MRGPRX2, protein kinase A, and PI3 kinase pathways is also rapid. Many unrelated drugs can activate the MRGPRX2 pathway, including neuromuscular blocking agents, quinolones, icatibant, polymyxin B, and phenothiazine. Certain opiates, notably codeine and morphine, directly activate mast cells via the protein kinase A and PI3 kinase pathways.[29]

The clinical symptoms associated with direct mast cell activation with NSAIDs typically take approximately 104 minutes to be apparent.[30] NSAIDs induce mast cells to release cycLTs and PGD2 and platelets to release PGD2. Boyce[15] reviewed the idiosyncratic activation of mast cells by nonselective COX inhibitors in 2019. He concluded that this intolerance is due to a complex multifactorial process that leads to dysregulation of mast cell function with an aberrant dependency on COX-1–derived prostaglandin E_2 to maintain homeostasis. Complement-derived anaphylatoxins, including C3a, C4a, and most importantly C5a, can also activate mast cells. C5a can also activate neutrophils. Iron nanoparticles can directly activate complement and intracellular Toll-like receptors 3, 7, and 9 and IL-1β.[27]

SMALL MOLECULES

Small molecules, in general, must be able to bind to autologous proteins to induce antigen-specific antibody production. Supposedly inert ingredients such as polyethoxylated castor oil derivatives including Kolliphor EL are present in a number of parenteral anticancer chemotherapeutics, vitamin K, and cyclosporin preparations. These materials can activate the complement system and directly activate mast cells.[31]

HUMAN AND HUMANIZED PROTEINS

The widely used anti–B-cell monoclonal rituximab is associated with high rates of adverse reactions, up to 77%, with initial exposure.[32] Most are only grade 1 or 2, but those with grade 3 or 4 reactions warrant a workup for immune-mediated hypersensitivity. Replacement recombinant proteins in individuals unable to make the protein commonly induce strong IgG immune responses that can also activate compliment and induce anaphylaxis.[33] IgE immune responses are also possible, but rarer.[33] With humanized monoclonal antibodies the rates of clinically significant IgG-mediated or IgE-mediated hypersensitivity is typically less than 5% with prolonged recurrent exposures.[34] With replacement proteins in individuals with a genetic inability to produce the protein, the rates are much higher, and approach 100% with recurrent exposures.[35] Antibodies are typically directed against protein epitopes on biologicals, but antibodies against carbohydrates, the classic case being alpha-gal, are also possible with therapeutic proteins.[36]

XENOGENEIC PROTEINS

The most common xenogeneic protein that individuals are exposed to during health care include latex, bovine serum albumin, and mouse monoclonal antibodies.[37,38] All are able to induce robust IgG immune responses with parenteral or mucosal exposures, and occasionally IgE responses resulting in anaphylaxis. With repeat exposures to xenogeneic proteins such as bovine serum albumin or mouse monoclonal antibodies, the rates of immunologically mediated adverse reactions are high and can also approach 100%.[38]

CONFIRMING IMMUNOLOGICALLY MEDIATED HYPERSENSITIVITY

In general, intradermal skin testing for injectable therapeutic proteins can be safely performed with the materials diluted to 1 μg/mL, using at least 7-mm wheel with flare > wheel as the criterion for a positive test result.[39] Small molecules used for diagnostic skin testing must be able to haptenate serum proteins and not be direct mast cell activators through non–IgE-mediated pathways.

For suspected T-cell–mediated hypersensitivity, a single challenge with a therapeutic dose followed by approximately 1 week of observation is adequate in most settings to confirm current tolerance.[5]

Before all challenges, it is essential to obtain informed consent from the patient.[5] The patient must be willing to experience a reaction at least a severe as the index reaction, and the physicians doing the testing must have the ability to treat any potential challenge reactions and follow the patient long enough based on the time to the onset of the index reaction and the suspected mechanism of the feared reaction.[5]

Stevenson and coworkers[40] reported in 2019 on a risk stratification strategy guiding penicillin allergy delabeling evaluations. They determined that any patient with a benign penicillin-associated rash more than 1 year ago could safely undergo a direct oral challenge with a therapeutic amoxicillin dose. We had previously come to the same conclusion.[21]

Krantz and coworkers[22] reported in 2019 on 204 individuals rechallenged with trimethoprim-sulfamethoxazole and noted only 13 (6.4%) were challenge positive. Younger age and short time since index reactions were associated with positive challenge reactions. We have noted that despite having a negative challenge, subsequent therapeutic exposure can still result in a 5% to 10% rate of recurrent reactions, although sometimes after tolerating several therapeutic courses. The key take-home message is that reactions are possible after all drug exposures, even after negative hypersensitivity testing.

MANAGING PATIENTS WITH HISTORICAL REACTIONS WITHOUT TESTING OR RECHALLENGE

Not all suspected immune-related or immune-mediated reactions require testing or diagnostic rechallenges. Radiocontrast hypersensitivity reactions are relatively rare with the non-ionic iso-osmolar radiocontrasts commonly used now, compared with hypertonic hyperosmolar media used historically.[41] Both delayed-onset apparent T-cell–mediated hypersensitivity, 2 to 5 days after exposure, and acute-onset direct mast cell activation, within minutes of exposure, can occur with non-ionic iso-osmolar radiocontrasts. Pretreatment with corticosteroids and antihistamines has not been shown to reduce recurrent acute-onset or delayed-onset reaction rates when the same material is administered in the future.[41] Most patients can be safely managed by just selecting an alternative non-ionic iso-osmolar radiocontrast.[41]

Slowing the infusion rate and pretreatment with NSAIDs and antihistamines will often reduce infusion-associated reactions with protein biologic therapeutics.[42]

DESENSITIZATIONS

Desensitization can be reliably accomplished only when IgE-mediated allergy has been confirmed and in a few other situations in which mast cell activation occurs via a non-IgE–mediated mechanism.[42] It is not possible to desensitize individuals with T-cell–mediated hypersensitivity, although it may be possible to treat through mild reactions.[5] The key to a successful desensitization is administering doubling doses of the material every 15 to 30 minutes, starting at below the threshold dose needed to initiate anaphylaxis, typically approximately 1/2000th of the therapeutic dose, and continuing up to the therapeutic dose. Castells and coworkers[42] have published a 3-bag protocol that works for both therapeutic proteins and small molecules. For medications that require sustained exposures, it is essential to maintain continuous exposure, or anaphylaxis may occur with repeat exposure. If an individual requires a medication acutely that requires a sustained exposure and had a positive diagnostic challenge reaction to a therapeutic dose, once the challenge reaction is treated and the patient is stabilized, it is appropriate to just continue the therapeutic dosing, maintaining constant exposure.

BLOCKING NEW IMMUNE REACTIONS

The use of replacement recombinant proteins for a variety of genetic diseases and adenovirus vectors in gene therapy has led to the need to be able to block new antibody production and new T-cell–mediated immune responses. Adenovirus vectors used for gene transfer therapies commonly induce a strong protective immune response, precluding reuse of the same vector.[26] It is important to test subjects before exposure to ensure they do not have a natural immunity to the vector.[26]

Currently the strategies used to prevent immune responses to biologic therapies are the same as those used for treating autoimmune diseases or with organ transplantation. These methods include suppression of autoantibody production with steroids or other immunosuppressive drugs, such as azathioprine, methotrexate, or by knocking out B cells that produce antibodies, such as the anti-CD20 antibody rituximab, and/or immunomodulation that targets T-cell function, such as cyclosporine or mycophenolate.[43]

The first report using engineered T cells against an autoreactive B-cell receptor/autoreactive B cells was in a preclinical model of pemphigus vulgaris in 2006.[44] In theory, one could specifically target autoreactive B cells and thus deplete circulating autoantibodies, although the approach has not proceeded into clinical trials to date.

B-cell depletion with rituximab has been widely used for some 20 years now to manage autoimmune conditions and B-cell malignancies. There is a certain degree of specificity in that autoantibodies appear to decline more than the bulk of protective antibodies, probably owing to being produced by short-lived plasma cells. However, from the start, the desire has been to remove autoantibodies specifically without impact on normal B-cell function. This turns out to be a very difficult task for antibodies like rheumatoid factors but may be easier for antibodies to local antigens like acetylcholine receptor. A recent review by Chang and colleagues[45] suggests that specific autoantibody deletion strategies may at last be feasible, thus potentially leading to a method to block antibiotic production against large-molecule biologic therapies.

Immunosuppressants are widely used in transplantation immunology, such as cyclosporine, tacrolimus, pimecrolimus, mycophenolate mofetil, cyclophosphamide, and/or azathioprine, and a variety of monoclonal antibodies including baksilizimab.[43] Combination therapy with rituximab, methotrexate, and intravenous gamma globulin (IVIg) has been used to blunt the generation of new antigen-specific immune responses to acid alfa glucosidase when giving enzyme replacement therapy in Pompe disease.[33] It is typically started concurrently with enzyme replacement therapy. Organ transplantation preconditioning protocols using IVIg replacement after plasmapheresis, with or without rituximab and thymoglobulin induction therapy, combined with tacrolimus, mycophenolate mofetil, and/or prednisone have also been considered to blunt the development of new immune responses against adenovirus gene transfer vectors.

PATHOLOGIC IMMUNE ACTIVATION

Therapeutic materials that interfere with normal immune regulation, most notably muromanab-CD3, alemtuzumab, and rituximab, have been implicated in triggering cytokine storm.[46] The primary symptoms of cytokine storm include fever, edema, erythema, fatigue, and nausea. Capillary leak can occur with endothelial damage leading to acute respiratory distress syndrome, cardiovascular shock, disseminated intervascular coagulation, and renal failure. The primary cytokines implicated include TNFα, interferon-α, IL-1β, and IL-2, IL-4, IL-6, IL-8, IL-10, and IL-12. Cytokine storm management typically relies on blunting the effect of the preceding mediators through the use of angiotensin-converting enzyme inhibitors, angiotensin II receptor blockers, gemfibrozil, NSAIDs, corticosteroids, IVIg, hemofiltration, anti–IL-6 (tocilizumab), and blocking C5a activity with anti–vitamin D binding protein antibodies.[47,48]

PATHOLOGIC IMMUNE SUPPRESSION

Both B cell and T cells can be adversely affected by therapeutic material used to treat allergic conditions. Hypogammaglobulinemia, sometimes irreversible, can occur after the use of anti–B-cell monoclonal antibodies, including rituximab and belimumab. Tyrosine kinase inhibitors, imatinib and dasatinib, along with commonly used immuno-suppressives, including corticosteroids and azathioprine, can cause hypogammaglobulinemia.[49]

SUMMARY

Biologic therapeutics and other agents used to treat immune-mediated hypersensitivity conditions can result in immune-related adverse drug reactions and immunologically mediated hypersensitivity. Time to onset and the nature of the reactions are the keys to determining potential mechanisms. Diagnostic testing and rechallenge may be useful, and in the specific setting of IgE-mediated allergy, desensitization in possible. It remains extremely difficult to stop antigen-specific antibody or T-cell–mediated responses once they have occurred without inducing generalized immune suppression.

CLINICAL CARE POINTS

- The immune system can be involved in adverse reactions associated with therapeutic agents used to treat immune-mediated hypersensitivity conditions.
- Immune-mediated hypersensitivity can occur when medications are able to haptenate autologous proteins, which then activate B cells to produce antibodies, directly or indirectly activate T cells, trigger the complement system, and/or directly activate mast cells.
- Therapeutic agents can also trigger the immune system, resulting in generalized activation or suppression, leading to adverse reactions.
- Some humans can make immunoglobulin (Ig)E against just about every humanized monoclonal antibody or therapeutic protein with a molecular weight on greater than 5000 kD. The rate is much higher with nonhumanized therapeutic proteins.
- You can only reliably desensitize individuals with clinically significant IgE-mediated allergy. You cannot desensitize individuals with clinically significant T-cell–mediated hypersensitivity.
- Skin testing to identify clinically significant IgE-mediated allergy is possible with all therapeutic proteins, but with only a very limited set of smaller molecules that can haptenate autologous proteins and do not directly activate cutaneous mast cells.

DISCLOSURE

E. Macy has received research grants to study drug allergy from ALK. He has served on data and safety monitoring boards for BioMarin and Audentes. He has performed consulting for Kalobios and Audentes. He is a member of the Ask an Expert Panel of the American Academy of Allergy, Asthma, and Immunology.

REFERENCES

1. Blumenthal KG, Park MA, Macy EM. Redesigning the allergy module of the electronic health record. Ann Allergy Asthma Immunol 2016;117:126–31.
2. Demoly P, Adkinson NF, Brockow K, et al. International consensus on drug allergy. Allergy 2014;69:420–37.
3. Wheatley LM, Plaut M, Schewaninger JM, et al. Report from the Nation Institute of Allergy and Infectious Disease workshop on drug allergy. J Allergy Clin Immunol 2015;136:262–71.e2.

4. Aberer W. A position paper on drug allergy-pinpointing problems rather than suggesting solutions. Allergy 2016;71:1079–80.
5. Macy E, Romano A, Khan D. Practical management of antibiotic hypersensitivity in 2017. J Allergy Clin Immunol Pract 2017;5:577–86.
6. Nel AE. T-cell activation through the antigen receptor. Part 1: Signaling components, signaling pathways, and signal integration at the T-cell antigen receptor synapse. J Allergy Clin Immunol 2002;109:758–70.
7. Pichler WJ, Adam J, Watkins S, et al. Drug hypersensitivity: How drugs stimulate T cells via pharmacological interaction with immune receptors. Int Arch Allergy Immunol 2015;168:13–24.
8. Chiriac AM, Macy E. Large health system databases and drug hypersensitivity. J Allergy Clin Immunol Pract 2019;7:2125–31.
9. Davis RL, Gallagher MA, Asgari MM, et al. Identification of Stevens-Johnson syndrome and toxic epidermal necrolysis in electronic health record databases. Pharmacoepidemiol Drug Saf 2015;24:684–92.
10. Pichler WJ. Adverse side-effects to biological agents. Allergy 2006;61:912–20.
11. Neftel KA, Walti M, Schulthess HK, et al. Adverse reactions following intravenous penicillin-G relate to degradation of the drug in vitro. Klin Wochenschr 1984; 62:25–9.
12. Blumenthal KG. The role of the clinical history in drug allergy prediction. J Allergy Clin Immunol Pract 2018;6:149–50.
13. Peter JP, Lehloenya R, Dlamini S, et al. Severe delayed cutaneous and systemic reactions to drugs: a global perspective on the science and art of current practice. J Allergy Clin Immunol Pract 2017;5:547–63.
14. Porebski G, Kwiecien K, Pawica M, et al. Mas-related G protein-coupled receptor-X2 (MRGPRX2) in drug hypersensitivity reactions. Front Immunol 2018;9:3027.
15. Boyce JA. Aspirin sensitivity: lessons in the regulation (and dysregulation) of mast cell function. J Allergy Clin Immunol 2019;144:875–81.
16. Bourgeols GP, Cafardi JA, Groysman V, et al. A review of DRESS-associated myocarditis. J Am Acad Dermatol 2012;66:e229–36.
17. Nakamura Y. Biomarkers for immune checkpoint inhibitor-mediated tumor response and adverse events. Front Med 2019;6:119.
18. Bajwa R, Cheema A, Khan T, et al. Adverse effects of immune checkpoint inhibitors (programmed death-1 inhibitors and cytotoxic T-lymphocyte-associated protein-4 inhibitors): results of a retrospective study. J Clin Med Res 2019;11: 225–36.
19. Calabrese L, Mariette X. Chronic inflammatory arthritis following checkpoint inhibitor therapy for cancer: game changing implications. Ann Rheum Dis 2020. https://doi.org/10.1136/anntheumdis-2019-216510.
20. Macy E, Ho NJ. Multiple drug intolerance syndrome: prevalence, clinical characteristics and management. Ann Allergy Asthma Immunol 2012;108:88–93.
21. Banks TA, Tucker M, Macy E. Evaluating penicillin allergies without skin testing. Curr Allergy Asthma Rep 2019;19:27.
22. Krantz MS, Stone CA, Abreo A, et al. Oral challenge with trimethoprim-sulfamethoxazole in patients with "sulfa" antibiotic allergy. J Allergy Clin Immunol Pract 2020;8(2):757–60.e4.
23. Macy E, Ho NJ. Adverse reactions associated with therapeutic antibiotic use after penicillin skin testing. Perm J 2011;15:31–7.
24. Macy E, Mangat R, Burchette RJ. Penicillin skin testing in advance of need: multiyear follow-up in 568 test result-negative subjects exposed to oral penicillins. J Allergy Clin Immunol 2003;111:1111–5.

25. Blumenthal KG, Li Y, Acker WW, et al. Multiple drug intolerance syndrome and multiple drug allergy syndrome: epidemiology and associations with anxiety and depression. Allergy 2018;73:2012–23.

26. Ahi YS, Bangari DS, Mittal SK. Adenoviral vector immunity: its implications and circumvention strategies. Curr Gene Ther 2011;11:307–20.

27. Verhoef JJF, de Groot AM, van Moorsel M, et al. Iron nanomedicines induce toll-like receptor activation, cytokine production and complement activation. Biomaterials 2017;119:68–77.

28. Finkelman FD, Khodoun MV, Strait R. Human IgE-independent systemic anaphylaxis. J Allergy Clin Immunol 2016;137:1674–80.

29. Sheen CH, Schleimer RP, Kulka M. Codeine induces human mast cell chemokine and cytokine production: Involvement of G-protein activation. Allergy 2007;62:532–8.

30. Woessner KM, White AA. Evidence-based approach to aspirin desensitization in aspirin-exacerbated respiratory disease. J Allergy Clin Immunol 2014;133:286–7.e1-9.

31. Renier R, Breynaert C, Dens AC, et al. Allergic reactions to polyethoxylated castor oil derivatives: a guide to decipher confusing names on pharmaceutical labels. Allergy Clin Immunol Pract 2020;8(3):1136–8.e2.

32. Levin AS, Otani IM, Lax T, et al. Reactions to rituximab in an outpatient infusion center: a 5-year review. Allergy Clin Immunol Pract 2017;5:107–13.

33. Banugaria SG, Prater SN, Patel TT, et al. Algorithm for the early diagnosis and treatment of patients with cross reactive immunologic material-negative classic infantile Pompe disease: a step toward improving efficacy of ERT. PLoS One 2013;8:e67052.

34. Bots S, Vande Casteele N, Brandse JF, et al. Antibody development against biologic agents used for the treatment of inflammatory bowel disease and antibody prevention with immunosuppressives. Cochrane Database Syst Rev 2016;(5):CD012147.

35. Rairkar M, Kazi ZB, Desai A, et al. High dose IVIG successfully reduces high rhGAA IgG antibody titers in a CRIM-negative infantile Pompe disease patient. Mol Genet Metab 2017;122:76–9.

36. Stone CA Jr, Choudhary S, Patterson MF, et al. Tolerance of porcine pancreatic enzymes despite positive skin testing in alpha-gal allergy. J Allergy Clin Immunol Pract 2020. https://doi.org/10.1016/j.jaip.2019.12.004.

37. Eck EK, Macy E, Huber W. Natural rubber latex protein allergy prevention and exposure control. Perm J 1998;2:15–8.

38. Macy E, Bulpitt K, Champlin RE, et al. Anaphylaxis to infusion of autologous bone marrow: an apparent reaction to self, mediated by IgE to bovine serum albumin. J Allergy Clin Immunol 1989;83:871–5.

39. Quirt JA, Wen X, Kim J, et al. Venom allergy testing: is a graded approach necessary? Ann Allergy Asthma Immunol 2016;116:49–51.

40. Stevenson B, Trevenen M, Klinken E, et al. Multicenter Australian study to determine criteria for low- and high-risk penicillin testing in outpatients. Allergy Clin Immunol Pract 2020;8(2):681–9.e3.

41. Macy EM. Current epidemiology and management of radiocontrast-associated acute- and delayed-onset hypersensitivity: a review of the literature. Perm J 2018;22:17–072.

42. Castells MC, Tennant NM, Sloane DE, et al. Hypersensitivity reactions to chemotherapy: outcomes and safety of rapid desensitization in 413 cases. J Allergy Clin Immunol 2008;122:574–80.

43. Zhang W, Chen D, Chen Z, et al. Successful kidney transplantation in highly sensitized patients. Front Med 2011;5:80–5.
44. Ellebrect CT, Bhoj VG, Nace A, et al. Reengineering chimeric antigen receptor T cells for targeted therapy of autoimmune disease. Science 2016;353:179–84.
45. Chang HD, Tokoyoda K, Hoyer B, et al. Pathogenic memory plasma cells in auto-immunity. Curr Opin Immunol 2019;61:86–91.
46. Zubiri L, Allen IM, Taylor MS, et al. Immune-related adverse events in the setting of PD-1/L1 inhibitor combination therapy. Oncologist 2019;25:1–7.
47. Gerlach H. Agents to reduce cytokine storm. F1000Res 2016;5(F1000 Faculty Rev):2909.
48. Simonaggio A, Michot JM, Voisin LA, et al. Evaluation of readministration of im-mune checkpoint inhibitors after immune-related adverse events in patient with cancer. JAMA Oncol 2019;5:1310–7.
49. Patel SY, Carbone J, Jolles S. The expanding field of secondary antibody defi-ciency: causes, diagnosis, and management. Front Immunol 2019;10:33.

Biologics for the Treatment of Allergic Conditions: Eosinophil Disorders

Bianca Olivieri, MD, Elisa Tinazzi, MD, PhD, Marco Caminati, MD,
Claudio Lunardi, MD*

KEYWORDS

- Eosinophils • Biologics • IL-5 • EGPA • HES • ABPA • EoE • CEP

KEY POINTS

- Interleukin (IL)-5 and IL-5 receptor are excellent therapeutic targets for eosinophil-associated diseases.
- Biologics have a steroid-sparing effect in eosinophil disorders.
- Mepolizumab added to glucocorticoids is useful in the relapse of nonsevere symptoms of eosinophilic granulomatosis with polyangiitis.
- Anti–IL-5 monoclonal antibodies are promising therapies for hypereosinophilic syndrome and chronic eosinophilic pneumonia, but further studies are needed.
- The role of biotechnological drugs in eosinophilic esophagitis and allergic bronchopulmonary aspergillosis is still uncertain.

INTRODUCTION

Inhibition of Interleukin 5 and Interleukin 5 Receptor in Eosinophil Disorders

Eosinophil-associated diseases are characterized by a common pathogenetic background, represented by eosinophilic inflammation and overexpression of IL-5.[1] Transgenic mice constitutively expressing the IL-5 gene develop blood eosinophilia and also have eosinophilic infiltrates in spleen, bone marrow, peritoneal exudate, lungs, lymph nodes, and gut lamina propria.[2,3] In support of this, IL-5–deficient mice (gene knockout), although they continue to produce basal eosinophil levels, do not develop blood or tissue eosinophilic response to helminth infection and lung damage, airways hyperreactivity, and remodeling in murine allergic asthma models.[4,5] These studies highlight the importance of the role of IL-5 in promoting the production and function of eosinophils in vivo. Moreover, the depletion of eosinophils does not seem to be associated with pathologic manifestations or specific abnormalities.[6] With these

Department of Medicine, University Hospital GB Rossi, University of Verona, Piazzale LA Scuro, 10, Verona 37134, Italy
* Corresponding author.
E-mail address: claudio.lunardi@univr.it

Immunol Allergy Clin N Am 40 (2020) 649–665
https://doi.org/10.1016/j.iac.2020.07.001
0889-8561/20/© 2020 Elsevier Inc. All rights reserved.

premises, it becomes evident that IL-5 and its receptor are excellent therapeutic targets for eosinophil-associated diseases. Three monoclonal antibodies (mAbs) targeting IL-5 currently are available on the market and approved for their use in severe asthma: mepolizumab and reslizumab block circulating IL-5,preventing the binding to its receptor,[7] whereas benralizumab binds to IL-5Ra. In addition, through its constant fragment crystallizable region, benralizumab binds to the FcgIIIRa receptor expressed by natural killer cells, thus inducing eosinophil apoptosis caused by the release of proapoptotic proteins, such as granzymes and perforins. This is the antibody-dependent cellular cytotoxicity (ADCC) mechanism induced by benralizumab against not only eosinophils but also, to a small extent, basophils.[8]

Anti–IL-5 mAbs also have been investigated, in addition to severe asthma, in many other eosinophil-associated diseases, such as eosinophilic granulomatosis with polyangiitis (EGPA), hypereosinophilic syndrome (HES), eosinophilic esophagitis (EoE), allergic bronchopulmonary aspergillosis (ABPA), and chronic eosinophilic pneumonia (CEP). This article discusses the evidence available so far, from case reports to clinical studies, on the use of biologics in eosinophil disorders.

Eosinophils

Eosinophils are white blood cells that are part, together with neutrophils and basophils, of the subgroup of granulocytes. They comprise approximately 200 large cytoplasmic granules, which contain mainly cytotoxic cationic proteins, including major basic protein 1 and 2, eosinophil cationic protein, eosinophil peroxidase, and eosinophil-derived neurotoxin.[9,10]

Eosinophils differentiate from a myeloid multipotent progenitor in bone marrow due to the interaction of transcription factors, including GATA-1 (a zinc family finger member), PU.1 (an ETS family member), and C/EBP members (CCAAT/enhancer-binding protein family). GATA-1 is the main factor that determines, in its presence, the differentiation into eosinophil and, in its absence, into macrophage or neutrophil. On the contrary, friend of GATA-1 (FOG-1) works as a coactivator of GATA-1, promoting the erythroid differentiation; therefore, it must be down-regulated for eosinophil development.[11] The differentiation of eosinophils is regulated by T-cell–derived cytokines and growth factors, such as interleukin (IL)-3, IL-5, and granulocyte-macrophage colony-stimulating factor (GM-CSF).[1] Of these cytokines, IL-5 is eosinophil-lineage specific and critical for terminal eosinophil differentiation. The surface expression of IL-5 receptor (IL-5R) is one of the terminal steps in eosinophil hematopoiesis.[12] Its expression promotes eosinophil activation and survival, making this receptor an attractive target for modulation of eosinophil levels.[10]

Physiologically, only a small number of eosinophils are released from the bone marrow, making up approximately 1% to 3% of white blood cells. In the blood stream, eosinophils persist for 18 hours to 24 hours, or even longer in conditions associated with blood eosinophilia, and then they migrate to extravascular sites.[13] In healthy subjects, eosinophils are present in the spleen, lymph nodes, and lower gastrointestinal tract but also in thymus, mammary glands, and uterus, where their physiologic functions still are not completely known.[14]

In cases of particular conditions, most frequently helminthic infections or allergic diseases, eosinophilopoiesis is increased by Helper T cell (T_H)2 cytokines, such as IL-3, IL-5, and GM-CSF. Once at the site of injury, eosinophils can release cytotoxic granule proteins, causing destruction of parasite infections if present and also inflammation and tissue damage. Eosinophils also can exacerbate the inflammatory response by releasing lipid mediators, including leukotriene C_4, platelet-activating factor, and liposins, and cytokines, such as IL-2, IL-4, IL-6, IL-10, and IL-12, which promote T-cell proliferation and activation and T_H1/T_H2 polarization.[9] Eosinophils can secrete transforming growth factor (TGF)-β and other molecules involved in tissue remodeling processes[15]; one example of this is the airway remodeling in eosinophilic asthma.[16] Activated eosinophils can interact with extracellular matrix components, especially fibronectin, and promote their own survival in the inflamed tissue by the autocrine secretion of IL-5, IL-3, and GM-CSF.[17,18] Furthermore, the harmful action of activated eosinophils is enhanced by other cells, including mast cells, basophils, T_H1, T_H17, and B cells.[19] Eosinophils also participate in the immune response by playing the role of antigen presenting cells: only after cytokine stimulation (IL-3, IL-4, GM-CSF, and interferon-γ), eosinophils express costimulatory molecules and major histocompatibility complex II molecules on the cell surface through which they expose a variety of processed antigens in order to stimulate T-lymphocyte responses.[20]

Interleukin-5

IL-5 initially was identified in mice as a B-cell growth and differentiation factor[21,22]; then it was understood that it corresponded to eosinophil differentiation factor, a lineage-specific cytokine for eosinophilopoiesis.[23] Further studies highlighted the effect of IL-5 also on basophils, but in any case its major role is on the eosinophils.[24]

IL-5 is produced, together with other T_H2 cytokines, such as IL-4, IL-13, and GM-CSF, mainly from T_H2 cells and innate lymphoid cells type 2[19] but also from B cells, mast cells, eosinophils, basophils, and epithelial cells.[25]

The IL-5R is expressed exclusively on eosinophils, basophils, and mouse B-cell precursors as well as mature B1 cells. It is composed of an alpha chain (IL-5Rα), which is specific for the IL-5 molecule, and a beta chain (β), which is shared by IL-13 and GM-CSF receptors and does not bind any ligand but participates in the signal transduction. The soluble form has an antagonistic effect on IL-5 signaling because it does not trigger the signal transduction. Monomeric forms of IL-5Rα have low affinity; instead, after dimerization with β chain, the affinity becomes higher.[26,27] When IL-5R binds its ligand, the JAK/STAT, MAPK, and PI-3K pathways are activated; MAPK pathway then activates nuclear factor kB and consequently eosinophilic/ T_H2 cytokines production.[28]

Therefore, IL-5 is responsible for eosinophils differentiation, maturation, and activation and for their tissue recruitment. This cytokine also is able to enhance eosinophils degranulation and antibody-dependent cytotoxicity[19–29] and prolong the eosinophils survival by inhibiting their apoptosis.[30]

Eosinophilic Granulomatosis with Polyangiitis

EGPA, previously known as Churg-Strauss syndrome, is one of the antineutrophil cytoplasmic antibodies (ANCA)-associated vasculitides. It is a necrotizing granulomatous vasculitis predominantly affecting small to medium vessels, associated with asthma, chronic rhinosinusitis, and eosinophilia.[31] It is a multisystem disorder characterized by lung involvement, which also is the most common feature, followed by cutaneous, cardiovascular, neurologic, renal, and gastrointestinal involvement. Characteristics of the disease are the presence of eosinophilic infiltrates in the internal organs and the presence of ANCA, although only in approximately 30% to 40% of the cases.[32]

The disease is characterized by 3 phases that can overlap each other and progress at varying intervals: asthma and other allergic symptoms, blood and tissue eosinophilia, and finally necrotizing vasculitis. Eosinophils are thought to play a major role in the pathogenesis of EGPA because they participate in all 3 stages of the disease, but the precise mechanism of eosinophil-mediated inflammation remains not completely understood. Organ damage can be caused by the direct action of eosinophils infiltrating the tissue and/or by the ischemic phenomenon due to the occlusion of small arteries by inflammatory cell infiltration or clotting.[33]

A diagnosis is based on 5 criteria established by the American College of Rheumatology: asthma, eosinophils higher than 10% on the differential leukocyte count, mononeuropathy (including multiplex) or polyneuropathy, migratory or transient pulmonary opacities, paranasal sinus abnormality, and biopsy containing a blood vessel wall rich in eosinophils. The presence of 4 or more criteria has a sensitivity of 85% and a specificity of 99.7% for EGPA.[34]

The cornerstone of EGPA therapy is systemic glucocorticoids, used as monotherapy or in combination with other immunosuppressive agents, such as cyclophosphamide, methotrexate, azathioprine, and mofetil mycophenolate, or with rituximab, an anti-CD20 mAb.[35] The therapeutic choice is guided by the type, the severity of organ involvement and by score systems, such as the 5-factor score (FFS).[36] Cyclophosphamide is indicated in the induction phase for severe cases and is the first choice for the cardiac involvement. Rituximab is the best choice in case of disease exacerbation, renal involvement, and ANCA-positive patients, because it obtains a more sustained response. The first large randomized study on the use of rituximab as induction-remission treatment in EGPA (REOVAS study, https://clinicaltrials.gov/ct2/show/NCT02807103) and also another phase III trial for its use in remission maintenance currently is under way (MAINRITSEG trial, https://clinicaltrials.gov/ct2/show/NCT03164473). After remission, the most used in the maintenance phase are methotrexate, azathioprine, or mofetil mycophenolate.[32,35,37]

Mepolizumab is the first anti–IL-5 mAb to be approved by the Food and Drug Administration (FDA) for the treatment of EGPA. It is used at a dose of 300 mg administered subcutaneously once every 4 weeks, which is higher than the dose of 100 mg every 4 weeks used for severe eosinophilic asthma. It has not yet been evaluated whether the 300-mg dose is superior in terms of efficacy than a dose of 100 mg.

Kahn and colleagues[38] reported the first case of refractory EGPA treated with mepolizumab: a 28-year-old woman who presented with a long history of asthma, hypereosinophilia (HE), myocarditis and interstitial pneumonia at onset. Over the years, she had many relapses, including neurologic involvement, requiring multiple therapeutic changes: methotrexate, interferon alfa, cyclophosphamide, intravenous immunoglobulins, and azathioprine, in combination with corticosteroids. Remission was obtained with a monthly dose of mepolizumab.

Subsequently a small open-label study conducted on 7 patients described the steroid-sparing effect of mepolizumab.[39] Another phase II open-label study evaluated the use of mepolizumab for remission induction in 10 patients affected by relapsing or refractory EGPA. This study showed disease remission and glucocorticoid reduction in most patients, with no relapse while on treatment with mepolizumab. Instead, 7 relapses occurred after switching to methotrexate for maintenance.[40,41]

The pivotal study that led to the approval of mepolizumab by the FDA is the MIRRA study, published by Wechsler and colleagues[42] in 2017. This is the first multicenter randomized, placebo-controlled, double-blind, parallel-group, phase 3 trial that enrolled 136 patients with relapsing/refractory EGPA, randomly assigned to receive 300-mg subcutaneous mepolizumab or placebo every 4 weeks for 52 weeks. Patients were on a stable dose of corticosteroids and immunosuppressant agents. Over the 52-week period, 28% of patients in the mepolizumab group achieved remission (Birmingham Vasculitis Activity Score = 0 and prednisone ≤4 mg/day) for at least 24 weeks compared with 3% of those in the placebo group (odds ratio [OR] 5.91; 95% CI, 2.68–13.03; $P<.001$). Moreover, there was a significantly higher percentage of patients in the mepolizumab group (32%) compared with those in the placebo group (3%) who achieved remission at both week 36 and week 48 (OR 16.74; 95% CI, 3.61–77.56; P<.001). A total of 47% of the participants in the mepolizumab group compared with 81% of the placebo group did not reach the remission; moreover, a higher eosinophil count was paralleled by a better response to mepolizumab. In addition, patients in the mepolizumab group had less relapse than those in the placebo group (annualized relapse rate: 1.14 mepolizumab vs 2.27 placebo; rate ratio 0.50; 95% CI, 0.36–0.70; P<.001), allowing a reduction in the dose of glucocorticoids.[42] A post hoc analysis of MIRRA study, in which a comprehensive definition of clinical benefit was applied, showed that a higher percentage of patients (78%–87%) had benefit from treatment with mepolizumab.[43] It remains unexplained, however, why in the study approximately half of patients treated with mepolizumab did not achieve remission. The investigators hypothesized that some vasculitic manifestations are not due to the action of eosinophils but rather to an irreversible damage that is refractory to anti–IL-5 treatment. Another possibility is that mepolizumab, although it reduces the eosinophils in the blood, is not able to decrease tissue eosinophils.[42]

In conclusion, the addition of mepolizumab to daily glucocorticoid therapy has proved useful in relapse of nonsevere symptoms, such as asthma and/or sinonasal disease, but there is no evidence of its efficacy in severe disease or in remission maintenance. Mepolizumab in maintenance phase appears to have a steroid-sparing effect and is effective in alleviating asthma and sinonasal symptoms of EGPA patients.

Studies on the use of reslizumab (https://clinicaltrials.gov/ct2/show/NCT02947945) and benralizumab (BITE study, https://clinicaltrials.gov/ct2/show/NCT03010436 and MANDARA study, https://clinicaltrials.gov/ct2/show/NCT04157348) in EGPA currently are under way.

Few data are available for the use of omalizumab, an anti-IgE mAb, in patients with EGPA. A retrospective chart review of 18 patients with EGPA who were treated with omalizumab showed improvement in asthma control and a steroid-sparing effect but no benefit on eosinophil count.[44] A case report describes the effectiveness of the association between rituximab, that led to a rapid control of the vasculitis component, and omalizumab, that was beneficial on asthma and bronchospasm during the rituximab infusion.[45]

Hypereosinophilic Syndrome

HES is characterized by HE (absolute eosinophil count [AEC] >1.5 × 10⁹/L in the peripheral blood on 2 examinations at least 1 month apart and/or pathologic confirmation of tissue HE) associated with organ damage and/or dysfunction due to eosinophil toxicity, once other causes of HE are excluded. The most common presenting symptoms are weakness and fatigue, cough, dyspnea, myalgias, fever, and rhinitis. Eosinophil-related organ manifestations usually are fibrosis (lung, heart, digestive tract, skin, and so forth), thromboembolism, cutaneous and mucosal signs and symptoms (erythema, angioedema, ulceration, pruritus, and eczema), and peripheral or central neuropathy with chronic or recurrent neurologic deficit. There are several variant types of HES: familial HES; myeloproliferative variants, associated with platelet-derived growth factor receptors A and B (PDGFRA and PDGFRB) and fibroblast growth factor receptor 1 (FGFR1) rearrangements, Janus kinase 2 (JAK2) mutation or factor interacting with PAPOLA and CPSF1 (FIP1L1)-PDGFRA fusion; T-cell lymphocytic variants (L-HES), characterized by aberrant IL-5–producing T cells; and idiopathic HES, diagnosed when no underlying cause is determined.[46,47]

The goal of therapy is to limit eosinophil-mediated organ damage. Defining whether PDGFR rearrangement is present is fundamental because this variant responds well to imatinib. If other genetic mutations are present, many therapies can be used, such as JAK-inhibitors or hydroxyurea for variants with JAK2 mutation, interferon-alpha, or chemotherapy. Systemic glucocorticoids are the cornerstone of therapy for all other cases of HES. In recent years, anti–IL-5 mAbs have been used to treat HES, although they have not yet been officially approved.[47]

In 2003 Plötz and colleagues[48] presented 3 cases of HES patients with eosinophilic dermatitis treated with mepolizumab with benefit. Two case reports described the efficacy of mepolizumab in treating children with FIP1L1-PDGFRA–negative HES.[49,50] Garrett and colleagues[51] performed an open-label trial in which 4 HES patients received intravenous mepolizumab (dose of 10 mg/kg, maximum 750 mg) every 4 weeks for 3 treatments. All patients experienced a decrease in blood eosinophilia by week 28, an improvement in their symptoms and also in forced expiratory volume in 1 second and in quality-of-life measurements.

Rothenberg and colleagues[52] evaluated the efficacy, safety, and steroid-sparing effect of mepolizumab in the largest randomized, double-blind, placebo-controlled trial carried out in HES patients. All of 85 patients enrolled were FIP1L1-PDGFRA negative and were treated only with prednisone (20–60 mg/day) to achieve stable clinical status and AEC less than 1000/μL. Patients received intravenous infusion of mepolizumab, 750 mg, or placebo every 4 weeks during a 36-week period, while the steroid dose was tapered. The primary endpoint, that is reduction of the prednisone dose to 10 mg or less per day for at least 8 consecutive weeks, was reached in 84% of patients in the mepolizumab group compared with 43% of placebo group (hazard ratio 2.90%; 95% CI, 1.59–5.26; $P<.001$), without increase in HES clinical activity. Moreover, AEC less than 600/μL for at least 8 consecutive weeks was achieved by 95% of patients in the mepolizumab group compared with 45% of the placebo group (hazard ratio 3.53; 95% CI, 1.94–6.45; $P<.001$). Serious AEs occurred in 7 patients in the mepolizumab group (14 events, including 1 death) and 5 patients receiving placebo (7 events), none of which was considered related to treatment. A subanalysis of this study examined patients with L-HES variant, confirmed by abnormal T-cell immunophenotype, receiving mepolizumab. There was no difference in the possibility to taper corticosteroids during mepolizumab therapy between patients with L-HES and those with a normal T-cell profile. A lower proportion of patients, however, with L-HES, maintained AEC less than 600/μL.[53] An open-label extension to the study published by Rothenberg and colleagues[52] confirmed the safety and steroid-sparing effect of mepolizumab even in the long term.[54]

A randomized, double-blind, placebo-controlled study that evaluates the efficacy and safety of mepolizumab, 300 mg subcutaneous, every 4 weeks for 32 weeks, compared with placebo in patients with HES recently has been concluded. The primary endpoint is the proportion of patients who experienced at least 1 HES flare during the treatment period (https://clinicaltrials.gov/ct2/show/study/NCT02836496).

In conclusion, mepolizumab seems effective in the treatment of HES and to obtain a steroid-sparing effect. The studies only evaluated, however, patients who were FIP1L1-PDGFRA negative, already on steroid therapy, and with stable disease. For this reason, there are no recommendations to use mepolizumab for patients affected by HES variants that are unresponsive to systemic corticosteroids, such as FIP1L1-PDGFRA positive, or for patients with acute presentations or who have not received steroid therapy. Mepolizumab currently is available for HES only in clinical trials or for compassionate use.

Although on smaller numbers, reslizumab has also been evaluated for the treatment of HES in a pilot study of 4 patients. Four participants with refractory HES or intolerant to conventional treatment were treated with a single intravenous 1-mg/kg dose of reslizumab. Two of 4 patients had a rapid decrease in AEC and an improvement of symptoms. Response was not predicted by serum IL-5 levels or presence of FIP1L1-PDGFRA. The clinical and hematologic response lasted for more than 30 days after the infusion but was associated with a rebound in AEC, preceded by a rise in serum IL-5, and a severe exacerbation in both subjects at 6 weeks to 8 weeks after treatment.[55] A case of L-HES[56] and a case of HES with eosinophilic dermatitis[57] effectively treated with reslizumab also have been reported.

Kuang and colleagues[58] presented a randomized, double-blind, placebo-controlled, phase 2 trial of benralizumab in HES. Twenty patients with FIP1L1-PDGFRA-negative HES and AEC greater than 1000/μL received 3 monthly subcutaneous injections of either benralizumab (at a dosage of 30 mg) or placebo, while receiving stable therapy. The primary endpoint of 50% reduction of AEC at week 12 was achieved by 90% of the benralizumab group compared with 30% of the placebo group ($P = .02$). The percentage of patients who had a hematologic and clinical response to benralizumab was 74% at week 48. This observed response rate is similar to those reported for glucocorticoid and mepolizumab treatment of this disorder. Only the clinical disease subtype appeared to be associated with the clinical response; 2 nonresponders patients had a myeloid variant of HES with JAK2 mutation and 3 patients who had relapses had the lymphoid variant, although a patient with the same clinical subtype had a sustained response. Moreover, the numbers of bone marrow eosinophils, eosinophil precursors, and blood and bone marrow basophils were significantly decreased at week 12 in all the patients in the benralizumab group. In 7 patients with gastrointestinal eosinophilia, the gastrointestinal biopsies revealed an almost total depletion of eosinophils at week 24. Eight patients had a constellation of symptoms (fever, chills, headache, nausea, and so forth) approximately 6 hours after the first dose; however, these symptoms did not occur at the subsequent doses. A reasonable explanation of this reaction is the ADCC mechanism, given the timing, the nature of the symptoms, and the presence of elevated lactate dehydrogenase levels.[58] Studies on the use of benralizumab in HES currently are under way (NATRON study, https://clinicaltrials.gov/ct2/show/NCT04191304 and https://clinicaltrials.gov/ct2/show/study/NCT02130882).

In conclusion, anti–IL-5 mAbs are promising therapies for HES but further studies are necessary to evaluate the timing of their use, especially in the remission maintenance phase.

Eosinophilic Esophagitis

EoE is a T_H2-mediated disease in which chronic eosinophil-rich inflammation causes symptoms of esophageal dysfunction. A diagnosis of EoE is based on the presence of greater than or equal to 15 eosinophils per high-power field (HPF) in esophageal biopsy.[59] The goal of therapy is symptom resolution, histopathologic improvement, and prevention of complications, such as stenosis. Conventional treatments are proton pump inhibitor, topical swallowed steroids, systemic steroids, elimination diets, and/or esophageal dilation. These therapeutic options, however, although effective, are not completely satisfactory for all patients; therefore, the use of biologic drugs has been introduced.[60]

Studies on mepolizumab in EoE have given conflicting results, so its role is still uncertain. The first study was published in 2006 by Stein and colleagues[61] and presented 4 EoE patients treated with monthly intravenous infusion of mepolizumab (maximum dosage 750 mg) for 3 months. All patients had a decrease of AEC ($P<.05$) and improvement of symptoms and quality of life. In 3 of 4 patients there also was an improvement in the endoscopic findings, in particular, esophageal eosinophilia. In a randomized, double-blind trial, 11 patients with active EoE were enrolled to receive 2 intravenous 750-mg doses of mepolizumab 1 week apart or placebo. Those not in remission (<5 peak eosinophils/HPF) after 8 weeks repeated the 2 doses 4 weeks apart. None of the patients achieved the primary endpoint of fewer than 5 eosinophils/HPF, but a marked reduction of mean esophageal eosinophilia ($P = .03$) was seen in the mepolizumab group compared with the placebo group. Moreover, a reduction in the expression of molecules associated with esophageal remodeling, such as TGF-β, was observed in the mepolizumab group. Symptoms and endoscopic findings did not significantly change during the treatment period.[62] Assa'ad and colleagues[63] performed a multicenter, double-blind, placebo-controlled trial enrolling 59 children with EoE who received intravenous mepolizumab every 4 weeks for 3 infusions, at a dose of either 0.55 mg/kg, 2.5 mg/kg, or 10 mg/kg, or placebo. Four weeks after the last infusion, only 8.8% of children reached the primary endpoint of a peak eosinophil counts less than 5/HPF. Reduced peak and mean eosinophil counts, to less than 20/HPF, were observed in 31.6% and 89.5% of children, respectively. Furthermore, there were no significant improvements in symptoms or endoscopic findings. A study is under way on mepolizumab in EoE, currently recruiting patients (https://clinicaltrials.gov/ct2/show/NCT03656380).

The role of reslizumab also remains uncertain, with only 1 pediatric population study currently available. This study enrolled 226 children and adolescents with EoE, who were randomized to receive reslizumab at 3 different doses (1 mg/kg, 2 mg/kg, and 3 mg/kg) or placebo for 4 months. Peak esophageal counts were reduced in all reslizumab groups compared with baseline and placebo; however, there were no significant differences in clinical symptoms or quality-of-life measures.[64] Another study is under way in the pediatric population (https://clinicaltrials.gov/ct2/show/results/NCT00635089).

To date, there are no studies on the use of benralizumab in EoE, but there is an ongoing trail on eosinophilic gastritis (https://clinicaltrials.gov/ct2/show/NCT03473977).

In addition to IL-5, other targets for EoE treatment were assessed with variable results. Omalizumab, an anti-IgE mAb, first was used in a trial of 9 patients with eosinophil-associated gastrointestinal disorders, 7 of whom had concomitant EoE. Patients received omalizumab every 2 weeks for 16 weeks, whereas the other therapies remained unchanged. Omalizumab was associated with a decrease in AEC and serum-free IgE as well as with an improvement of symptoms. There also was a reduction in gastric and duodenal eosinophilia, but it did not reach statistical significance; moreover, esophageal eosinophilia remained unaffected.[65] Cases of 2 young EoE patients treated with omalizumab also have been reported. They experienced an improvement in symptoms but no improvement was seen in esophageal eosinophilia and endoscopic findings.[66] In a prospective, randomized, double-blind trial, 30 patients were randomized to receive either omalizumab or placebo every 2 weeks to 4 weeks for 16 weeks. Also in this study, omalizumab did not lead to an improvement in eosinophil counts in esophageal biopsies compared with placebo.[67] In a pilot study, 15 patients with long-standing EoE were treated with omalizumab for 12 weeks. After this period, only 33% of patients reached the remission, defined as histologic and clinical, and these patients were characterized by a low AEC value.[68]

Dupilumab is an mAb that binds IL-4Rα, thus inhibiting the IL-4 and IL-13 pathways, and currently is approved by FDA for atopic dermatitis, severe asthma, and chronic rhinosinusitis with nasal polyposis.[69] In a recent phase 2 trial, 47 adults with active EoE were randomized to receive weekly subcutaneous injections of dupilumab, at a dose of 300 mg, or placebo, for 12 weeks. Dupilumab obtained a significant improvement in dysphagia, endoscopic findings, and esophageal eosinophilia compared with placebo. Side effects, such as injection-site erythema and nasopharyngitis, were more common in the dupilumab group.[70] Trials currently are under way on the use of dupilumab in EoE (https://clinicaltrials.gov/ct2/show/NCT03633617) and in eosinophilic gastritis (https://clinicaltrials.gov/ct2/show/NCT03678545).

IL-13, another T_H2 cytokine, recently has been studied as a therapeutic target for EoE. Two anti–IL-13 mAbs, QAX576[71] and RPC4046,[72] have been used in patients with EoE with promising results.

Allergic Bronchopulmonary Aspergillosis

ABPA is a complex pulmonary disorder that occurs almost exclusively in patients with asthma or cystic fibrosis and is characterized by asthmatic symptoms, mucus plugging, pulmonary opacities, bronchiectasis, lung fibrosis, elevated AEC and total serum IgE, and detectable serum IgE or precipitating serum antibodies against *Aspergillus fumigatus* or aspergillus skin test positivity. It is the result of hypersensitivity reaction in response to colonization of the airways with *Aspergillus fumigatus*. An intense inflammatory T_H2 response thus is generated, with the production of IL-4, IL-5, and IL-13, which also cause the increase in blood and airway eosinophils and IgE. ABPA therapy consists of systemic and inhaled glucocorticoids and antifungal therapy (itraconazole or voriconazole).[73,74]

In order to reduce the use of corticosteroids and their long-term side effects, the introduction of an anti-IgE agent into ABPA therapy was evaluated. From the first published case of omalizumab used in ABPA,[75] many case reports have been described and these cases were collected in a systematic review in 2017. From the 102 cases analyzed, it emerged that omalizumab, most commonly administered 375 mg every 2 weeks, not only provided an important reduction in serum IgE, exacerbation rates, and steroid requirement but also improved pulmonary function parameters. There were no significant reported adverse events.[76] In an open-label study, 16 ABPA patients without cystic fibrosis were treated with omalizumab for 1 year and experienced a significant reduction in asthma exacerbations and in oral glucocorticoid dose compared with the year prior to start omalizumab.[77] In a randomized, placebo-controlled, crossover trial, 13 patients with ABPA and poorly controlled asthma were randomly assigned to monthly subcutaneous omalizumab, 750 mg, or placebo for 4 months, followed by a 3-month washout phase and then crossover to the opposite treatment. During the treatment period, the use of omalizumab was associated with a reduction in exacerbations and in fractional exhaled nitric oxide (FeNO) levels.[78] Some case series report promising results with omalizumab also in patients with ABPA associated with cystic fibrosis,[79,80] even if a double-blind, randomized, placebo-controlled study evaluating the safety and efficacy of omalizumab in patients with ABPA and cystic fibrosis has been stopped due to significant dropout rate of the patients (https://clinicaltrials.gov/ct2/show/results/NCT00787917).

To date, the effect of mepolizumab in ABPA has been evaluated only in case reports. In the 4 cases described, mepolizumab was administered at a dose of 100 mg every 4 weeks with the result of a significant improvement in asthmatic symptoms, lung function, chest radiograph images, and peripheral eosinophil count, allowing sparing of oral corticosteroids.[81–83] A case report described a patient with ABPA who was switched from omalizumab to mepolizumab. The patient was treated first with omalizumab (600 mg every 2 weeks), which improved her asthmatic symptoms but not the radiological findings and coexisting eosinophilic sinusitis and otitis media. After switching to mepolizumab (100 mg every 4 weeks), she experienced the resolution of these manifestations and the normalization of the eosinophil count.[84] Another case report described the use of omalizumab in combination with mepolizumab in a patient with ABPA in poor disease control when treated only with omalizumab. This combination made it possible to reduce the systemic corticosteroid dose and led to an improvement in symptoms but not in lung function.[85]

There currently is no evidence on the use of reslizumab in ABPA and only 3 cases have been described on the use of benralizumab. In the first, a 60-year-old patient was treated successfully with benralizumab, observing an improvement in chest images and peripheral eosinophil level after 1 month of treatment.[86] Tomomatsu and colleagues[87] recently published 2 cases of ABPA treated with mepolizumab and then switched to benralizumab, resulting in clearance of mucus plugs and a further decrease in the peripheral blood eosinophil count. A trial currently is under way on the use of benralizumab in ABPA (https://clinicaltrials.gov/ct2/show/NCT04108962).

Chronic Eosinophilic Pneumonia

CEP is a rare lung disease characterized by concomitant systemic and local eosinophilia, associated with bilateral lung infiltrates. The most common symptoms are prolonged cough and dyspnea. Most patients with CEP also have an allergic disease, such as asthma, atopic dermatitis, and allergic rhinitis. Elevated IgE levels, blood and tissue eosinophilia, and eosinophilia on bronchoalveolar lavage (BAL) are key elements of CEP. Therapy consists of systemic corticosteroids, usually with a good response. Inhaled corticosteroids also are used because patients frequently have comorbid asthma. Approximately 50% of patients have a relapse during tapering and/or after discontinuation of corticosteroid treatment; therefore, other therapies, such as biotechnological drugs, are needed in these phases.[88]

The first case report on the use of mepolizumab in CEP was published in 2018: a 65-year-old patient with CEP had a relapse after discontinuation of systemic corticosteroid therapy; he was started on mepolizumab, 100 mg, monthly instead of reintroducing corticosteroids. Approximately 1 month after the beginning of the treatment, his symptoms disappeared and AEC decreased to a normal level. After 3 months, there was a complete regression of parenchymal abnormalities at CT scan. The patient continued mepolizumab therapy without evidence of new relapses.[89] Another case report described the efficacy of mepolizumab in reducing symptoms, AEC, oxygen, and corticosteroid therapies and also in improving lung infiltrates on CT and lung function parameters in a patient already treated with omalizumab without beneficial effects.[90] An open-label retrospective study on the treatment of 10 patients with relapsing CEP with mepolizumab recently has been published. Subcutaneous mepolizumab was initiated, at a dose of 100 mg every 4 weeks, in 6 patients (approved dose in asthma), whereas 4 patients received 300 mg every 4 weeks (dose used in HES and EGPA). When they started treatment with mepolizumab, 7 of 10 patients were still receiving oral glucocorticoids and 5 patients inhaled corticosteroids for concomitant asthma. During the 9 months of follow-up, no side effects related to mepolizumab were recorded. Mepolizumab was associated with a significant reduction of relapses ($P = .002$) and of oral corticosteroids use. After 3 months of treatment, AEC significantly decreased and after 6 months there was a complete disappearance of lung lesions in 7 of 8 patients who underwent a CT scan.[91]

There currently are no reports in the literature on the use of reslizumab in CEP. As for benralizumab, a case report recently has been published. This is a 58-year-old woman with refractory CEP complicated with uncontrolled asthma, treated with a single 30-mg dose of benralizumab, without corticosteroid therapy. At 2 weeks, resolution of the patient's symptoms and of lung lesions at chest radiography were observed and lasted for 8 weeks. There also was a decrease in AEC and FeNO but no improvement in pulmonary function tests.[92] A case of a patient with a long history of relapsing CEP treated first with mepolizumab and then with benralizumab with benefit also has been reported.[93]

Omalizumab seems successful in case reports of CEP with prolonged dependence on systemic glucocorticoids, in association with positive skin tests for perennial allergens and elevated IgE levels.[94–96] The use of omalizumab in a patient with a very severe form of CEP has allowed her to be removed from the lung transplant waiting list, due to the significant improvement in her lung function after 24 months of treatment.[97]

There is only 1 reported case of CEP as a possible severe side effect of dupilumab. A 56-year-old patient with eosinophilic severe asthma was treated with dupilumab and after the tenth injection he presented a worsening of symptoms, increased AEC, and bilateral pulmonary thickening. BAL and transbronchial lung biopsy confirmed the diagnosis of CEP, which resolved after a prolonged treatment with oral corticosteroids.[98]

These biologics, especially omalizumab and mepolizumab, appear to be promising for reducing or discontinuing corticosteroid therapy in relapsing CEP cases. Randomized studies are needed, however, to confirm their efficacy and safety as well as to identify the best maintenance schedule.

CONCLUSION

mAbs enable acting against a precise molecular target, which often represents a key element in the pathogenesis of the disease, such as IL-5, in the case of eosinophil-associated diseases. The introduction of these new therapies allows avoiding the side effects derived from the long-standing use of corticosteroids, hitherto considered the cornerstone of therapy for eosinophilic diseases. Biologicals represent the first step toward precision medicine and in the not too distant future they will become an integral part of conventional therapies. To date, however, randomized clinical trials are needed to confirm the efficacy and safety of mAbs in large numbers of patients.

CLINICS CARE POINTS

- Eosinophil-associated diseases are characterized by eosinophilic inflammation and overexpression of IL-5. mAbs targeting IL-5, which currently are available for severe asthma, are being studied for eosinophilic diseases.
- Mepolizumab (anti-IL-5 mAb) has been approved by FDA for the treatment of EGPA at a dose of 300 mg administered subcutaneously once every 4 weeks. Mepolizumab added to glucocorticoid therapy is useful in EGPA relapse of non-severe symptoms, such as asthma and/or sinonasal disease, but there is no evidence of its efficacy in severe disease or in remission maintenance.
- The safety and steroid-sparing effect of mepolizumab, even in the long term, has been proved in patients with FIP1L1-PDGFRA–negative HES with stable disease. There are no recommendations, however, to use mepolizumab in patients who are nonresponders to systemic corticosteroids, such as FIP1L1-PDGFRA–positive variants, or in patients with acute presentations or who are naïve from steroid therapy. Benralizumab also is a promising therapy for HES, but further studies are needed.
- Studies on omalizumab (anti-IgE mAb), mepolizumab, and reslizumab (anti–IL-5 mAb) in EoE have given conflicting results, so their role in this situation remains uncertain. Dupilumab, an anti–IL-4Rα mAb that inhibits IL-4 and IL-13, and 2 other anti–L-13 mAbs have been used in patients with EoE with promising results.

- In ABPA, omalizumab improves pulmonary function parameters and obtains an important reduction in serum IgE, in exacerbation rates, and In steroid requirement. The effect of benralizumab and mepolizumab in ABPA has been evaluated only in case reports.
- In CEP, mepolizumab was evaluated in few patients with promising results. It was associated with a significant reduction of relapses, of oral corticosteroids use, and AEC and with an improvement of lung lesions at CT scan. Also, omalizumab seems promising in reducing corticosteroid therapy in relapsed CEP cases.

DISCLOSURE

The authors have nothing to disclose.

REFERENCES

1. Ackerman SJ, Bochner BS. Mechanisms of eosinophilia in the pathogenesis of hypereosinophilic disorders. Immunol Allergy Clin North Am 2007;27(3):357–75.
2. Dent LA, Strath M, Mellor AL, et al. Eosinophilia in transgenic mice expressing interleukin 5. J Exp Med 1990;172(5):1425–31.
3. Tominaga A, Takaki S, Koyama N, et al. Transgenic mice expressing a B cell growth and differentiation factor gene (interleukin 5) develop eosinophilia and autoantibody production. J Exp Med 1991;173(2):429–37.
4. Kopf M, Brombacher F, Hodgkin PD, et al. IL-5-deficient mice have a developmental defect in CD5+ B-1 cells and lack eosinophilia but have normal antibody and cytotoxic T cell responses. Immunity 1996;4(1):15–24.
5. Foster PS, Hogan SP, Ramsay AJ, et al. Interleukin 5 deficiency abolishes eosinophilia, airways hyperreactivity, and lung damage in a mouse asthma model. J Exp Med 1996;183(1):195–201.
6. Gleich GJ, Klion AD, Lee JJ, et al. The consequences of not having eosinophils. Allergy 2013;68(7):829–35.
7. Caminati M, Menzella F, Guidolin L, et al. Targeting eosinophils: severe asthma and beyond. Drugs Context 2019;8:1–15.
8. Pelaia C, Calabrese C, Vatrella A, et al. Benralizumab: From the basic mechanism of action to the potential use in the biological therapy of severe eosinophilic asthma. Biomed Res Int 2018;2018. https://doi.org/10.1155/2018/4839230.
9. Rothenberg ME, Hogan SP. The eosinophil. Annu Rev Immunol 2006;24(1): 147–74.
10. Riaz N, Wolden SL, Gelblum DY, et al. Eosinophils in mucosal immune responses. Mucosal Immunol 2016;118(24):6072–8.
11. Yamaguchi Y, Nishio H, Kishi K, et al. C/EBPβ and GATA-1 synergistically regulate activity of the eosinophil granule major basic protein promoter: Implication for C/EBPβ activity in eosinophil gene expression. Blood 1999;94(4):1429–39.
12. Clutterbuck E, Hirst E, Sanderson C. Human interleukin-5 (IL-5) regulates the production of eosinophils in human bone marrow cultures: comparison and interaction with IL-1, IL-3, IL-6, and GMCSF. Blood 1989;73(6):1504–12.
13. Uhm TG, Kim BS, Chung Y. Eosinophil development, regulation of eosinophil-specific genes, and role of eosinophils in the pathogenesis of asthma. Allergy Asthma Immunol Res 2012;4(2):68–79.
14. Roufosse F, Weller PF. Practical approach to the patient with hypereosinophilia. J Allergy Clin Immunol 2010;126(1):39–44.
15. Wong D, Elovic A, Matossian K, et al. Eosinophils from patients with blood eosinophilia express transforming growth factor beta 1. Blood 1991;78(10):2702–7.

16. Flood-Page P, Menzies-Gow A, Phipps S, et al. Anti-IL-5 treatment reduces deposition of ECM proteins in the bronchial subepithelial basement membrane of mild atopic asthmatics. J Clin Invest 2003;112(7):1029–36.

17. Anwar AR. Adhesion to fibronectin prolongs eosinophil survival. J Exp Med 1993; 177(3):839–43.

18. Walsh GM. Eosinophil Apoptosis and Clearance in Asthma. J Cell Death 2013; 6(1). https://doi.org/10.4137/JCD.S10818.

19. Morita H, Moro K, Koyasu S. Innate lymphoid cells in allergic and nonallergic inflammation. J Allergy Clin Immunol 2016;138(5):1253–64.

20. Shi H. Eosinophils function as antigen-presenting cells. J Leukoc Biol 2004;76(3): 520–7.

21. McKenzie DT, Filutowicz HI, Swain SL, et al. Purification and partial sequence analysis of murine B cell growth factor II (interleukin 5). J Immunol 1987;139(8): 2661–8.

22. Baumann MA, Paul CC. Interleukin-5 and Human B Lymphocytes. Methods 1997; 11(1):88–97.

23. Campbell HD, Tucker WQ, Hort Y, et al. Molecular cloning, nucleotide sequence, and expression of the gene encoding human eosinophil differentiation factor (interleukin 5). Proc Natl Acad Sci U S A 1987;84(19):6629–33.

24. Denburg J, Silver J, Abrams J. Interleukin-5 is a human basophilopoietin: induction of histamine content and basophilic differentiation of HL-60 cells and of peripheral blood basophil-eosinophil progenitors. Blood 1991;77(7):1462–8.

25. Caminati M, Pham D Le, Bagnasco D, et al. Type 2 immunity in asthma. World Allergy Organ J 2018;11:13.

26. Tavernier J, Devos R, Cornelis S, et al. A human high affinity interleukin-5 receptor (IL5R) is composed of an IL5-specific alpha chain and a beta chain shared with the receptor for GM-CSF. Cell 1991;66(6):1175–84.

27. Geijsen N, Leo Koenderman PJC. Specificity in cytokine signal transduction: lessons learned from the IL-3/IL-5/GM-CSF receptor family. Cytokine Growth Factor Rev 2001;12(1):19–25.

28. Rossjohn J, McKinstry WJ, Woodcock JM, et al. Structure of the activation domain of the GM-CSF/IL-3/IL-5 receptor common β-chain bound to an antagonist. Blood 2000;95(8):2491–8.

29. Sriaroon P, Ballow M. Biological modulators in eosinophilic diseases. Clin Rev Allergy Immunol 2016;50(2):252–72.

30. Yamaguchi Y, Suda T, Ohta S, et al. Analysis of the survival of mature human eosinophils: interleukin-5 prevents apoptosis in mature human eosinophils. Blood 1991;78(10):2542–7.

31. Jennette JC, Falk RJ, Bacon PA, et al. 2012 Revised International Chapel Hill consensus conference nomenclature of vasculitides. Arthritis Rheum 2013; 65(1):1–11.

32. Vega Villanueva KL, Espinoza LR. Eosinophilic vasculitis. Curr Rheumatol Rep 2020;22(1):5.

33. Khoury P, Grayson PC, Klion AD. Eosinophils in vasculitis: characteristics and roles in pathogenesis. Nat Rev Rheumatol 2014;10(8):474–83.

34. Masi AT, Hunder GG, Lie JT, et al. The American College of Rheumatology 1990 criteria for the classification of churg-strauss syndrome (allergic granulomatosis and angiitis). Arthritis Rheum 2010;33(8):1094–100.

35. Yates M, Watts RA, Bajema IM, et al. EULAR/ERA-EDTA recommendations for the management of ANCA-associated vasculitis. Ann Rheum Dis 2016;75(9): 1583–94.

36. Guillevin L, Pagnoux C, Seror R, et al. The five-factor score revisited. Medicine (Baltimore) 2011;90(1):19–27.
37. Emejuaiwe N. Treatment strategies in ANCA-associated vasculitis. Curr Rheumatol Rep 2019;21(7):33.
38. Kahn J-E, Grandpeix-Guyodo C, Marroun I, et al. Sustained response to mepolizumab in refractory Churg-Strauss syndrome. J Allergy Clin Immunol 2010; 125(1):267–70.
39. Kim S, Marigowda G, Oren E, et al. Mepolizumab as a steroid-sparing treatment option in patients with Churg-Strauss syndrome. J Allergy Clin Immunol 2010; 125(6):1336–43.
40. Moosig F, Gross WL, Herrmann K, et al. Targeting Interleukin-5 in Refractory and Relapsing Churg–Strauss Syndrome. Ann Intern Med 2011;155(5):341.
41. Herrmann K, Gross WL, Moosig F. Extended follow-up after stopping mepolizumab in relapsing/refractory Churg-Strauss syndrome. Clin Exp Rheumatol 2012;30(1 Suppl 70):S62–5. Available at: http://www.ncbi.nlm.nih.gov/pubmed/22512988.
42. Wechsler ME, Akuthota P, Jayne D, et al. Mepolizumab or placebo for eosinophilic granulomatosis with polyangiitis. N Engl J Med 2017;376(20):1921–32.
43. Steinfeld J, Bradford ES, Brown J, et al. Evaluation of clinical benefit from treatment with mepolizumab for patients with eosinophilic granulomatosis with polyangiitis. J Allergy Clin Immunol 2019;143(6):2170–7.
44. Celebi Sozener Z, Gorgulu B, Mungan D, et al. Omalizumab in the treatment of eosinophilic granulomatosis with polyangiitis (EGPA): single-center experience in 18 cases. World Allergy Organ J 2018;11(1):39.
45. Aguirre-Valencia D, Posso-Osorio I, Bravo J-C, et al. Sequential rituximab and omalizumab for the treatment of eosinophilic granulomatosis with polyangiitis (Churg-Strauss syndrome). Clin Rheumatol 2017;36(9):2159–62.
46. Valent P, Klion AD, Horny H-P, et al. Contemporary consensus proposal on criteria and classification of eosinophilic disorders and related syndromes. J Allergy Clin Immunol 2012;130(3):607–12.e9.
47. Shomali W, Gotlib J. World Health Organization-defined eosinophilic disorders: 2019 update on diagnosis, risk stratification, and management. Am J Hematol 2019;94(10):1149–67.
48. Plötz SG, Simon HU, Darsow U, et al. Use of an anti-interleukin-5 antibody in the hypereosinophilic syndrome with eosinophilic dermatitis. N Engl J Med 2003; 349(24):2334–9.
49. Mehr S, Rego S, Kakakios A, et al. Treatment of a Case of Pediatric Hypereosinophilic Syndrome with Anti-Interleukin-5. J Pediatr 2009;155(2):289–91.
50. Armoni Domany K, Shiran SI, Adir D, et al. The effect of mepolizumab on the lungs in a boy with hypereosinophilic syndrome. Am J Respir Crit Care Med 2020. https://doi.org/10.1164/rccm.201907-1376IM.
51. Garrett JK, Jameson SC, Thomson B, et al. Anti–interleukin-5 (mepolizumab) therapy for hypereosinophilic syndromes☆. J Allergy Clin Immunol 2004;113(1): 115–9.
52. Rothenberg ME, Klion AD, Roufosse FE, et al. Treatment of Patients with the Hypereosinophilic Syndrome with Mepolizumab. N Engl J Med 2008;358(12): 1215–28.
53. Roufosse F, de Lavareille A, Schandené L, et al. Mepolizumab as a corticosteroid-sparing agent in lymphocytic variant hypereosinophilic syndrome. J Allergy Clin Immunol 2010;126(4):828–35.e3.

54. Roufosse FE, Kahn J-E, Gleich GJ, et al. Long-term safety of mepolizumab for the treatment of hypereosinophilic syndromes. J Allergy Clin Immunol 2013;131(2): 461–7.e5.

55. Klion AD, Law MA, Noel P, et al. Safety and efficacy of the monoclonal anti–interleukin-5 antibody SCH55700 in the treatment of patients with hypereosinophilic syndrome. Blood 2004;103(8):2939–41.

56. Buttgereit T, Bonnekoh H, Church MK, et al. Effective treatment of a lymphocytic variant of hypereosinophilic syndrome with reslizumab. J Dtsch Dermatol Ges 2019;17(11):1171–2.

57. Kuruvilla M. Treatment of hypereosinophilic syndrome and eosinophilic dermatitis with reslizumab. Ann Allergy Asthma Immunol 2018;120(6):670–1.

58. Kuang FL, Legrand F, Makiya M, et al. Benralizumab for PDGFRA-negative hypereosinophilic syndrome. N Engl J Med 2019;380(14):1336–46.

59. Dellon ES, Liacouras CA, Molina-Infante J, et al. Updated International consensus diagnostic criteria for eosinophilic esophagitis: proceedings of the AGREE conference. Gastroenterology 2018;155(4):1022–33.e10.

60. Choudhury S, Baker S. Eosinophilic esophagitis: the potential role of biologics in its treatment. Clin Rev Allergy Immunol 2019. https://doi.org/10.1007/s12016-019-08749-6.

61. Stein ML, Collins MH, Villanueva JM, et al. Anti-IL-5 (mepolizumab) therapy for eosinophilic esophagitis. J Allergy Clin Immunol 2006;118(6):1312–9.

62. Straumann A, Conus S, Grzonka P, et al. Anti-interleukin-5 antibody treatment (mepolizumab) in active eosinophilic oesophagitis: a randomised, placebo-controlled, double-blind trial. Gut 2010;59(01):21–30.

63. Assa'ad AH, Gupta SK, Collins MH, et al. An antibody against IL-5 reduces numbers of esophageal intraepithelial eosinophils in children with eosinophilic esophagitis. Gastroenterology 2011;141(5):1593–604.

64. Spergel JM, Rothenberg ME, Collins MH, et al. Reslizumab in children and adolescents with eosinophilic esophagitis: Results of a double-blind, randomized, placebo-controlled trial. J Allergy Clin Immunol 2012;129(2):456–63.e3.

65. Foroughi S, Foster B, Kim N, et al. Anti-IgE treatment of eosinophil-associated gastrointestinal disorders. J Allergy Clin Immunol 2007;120(3):594–601.

66. Rocha R, Vitor AB, Trindade E, et al. Omalizumab in the treatment of eosinophilic esophagitis and food allergy. Eur J Pediatr 2011;170(11):1471–4.

67. Clayton F, Fang JC, Gleich GJ, et al. Eosinophilic esophagitis in adults is associated with IgG4 and not mediated by IgE. Gastroenterology 2014;147(3):602–9.

68. Loizou D, Enav B, Komlodi-Pasztor E, et al. A pilot study of omalizumab in eosinophilic esophagitis. Unutmaz D, ed. PLoS One 2015;10(3):e0113483.

69. Pesek RD, Gupta SK. Future therapies for eosinophilic gastrointestinal disorders. Ann Allergy Asthma Immunol 2020;124(3):219–26.

70. Hirano I, Dellon ES, Hamilton JD, et al. Efficacy of Dupilumab in a phase 2 randomized trial of adults with active eosinophilic esophagitis. Gastroenterology 2020;158(1):111–22.e10.

71. Rothenberg ME, Wen T, Greenberg A, et al. Intravenous anti–IL-13 mAb QAX576 for the treatment of eosinophilic esophagitis. J Allergy Clin Immunol 2015;135(2): 500–7.

72. Hirano I, Collins MH, Assouline-Dayan Y, et al. RPC4046, a monoclonal antibody against IL13, reduces histologic and endoscopic activity in patients with eosinophilic esophagitis. Gastroenterology 2019;156(3):592–603.e10.

73. Agarwal R, Sehgal IS, Dhooria S, et al. Developments in the diagnosis and treatment of allergic bronchopulmonary aspergillosis. Expert Rev Respir Med 2016; 10(12):1317–34.

74. Patel G, Greenberger PA. Allergic bronchopulmonary aspergillosis. Allergy Asthma Proc 2019;40(6):421–4.

75. van der Ent CK, Hoekstra H, Rijkers GT. Successful treatment of allergic bronchopulmonary aspergillosis with recombinant anti-IgE antibody. Thorax 2007;62(3): 276–7.

76. Li J-X, Fan L-C, Li M-H, et al. Beneficial effects of Omalizumab therapy in allergic bronchopulmonary aspergillosis: A synthesis review of published literature. Respir Med 2017;122(507):33–42.

77. Tillie-Leblond I, Germaud P, Leroyer C, et al. Allergic bronchopulmonary aspergillosis and omalizumab. Allergy 2011;66(9):1254–6.

78. Voskamp AL, Gillman A, Symons K, et al. Clinical efficacy and immunologic effects of omalizumab in allergic bronchopulmonary aspergillosis. J Allergy Clin Immunol Pract 2015;3(2):192–9.

79. Tanou K, Zintzaras E, Kaditis AG. Omalizumab therapy for allergic bronchopulmonary aspergillosis in children with cystic fibrosis: A synthesis of published evidence. Pediatr Pulmonol 2014;49(5):503–7.

80. Perisson C, Destruys L, Grenet D, et al. Omalizumab treatment for allergic bronchopulmonary aspergillosis in young patients with cystic fibrosis. Respir Med 2017;133:12–5.

81. Terashima T, Shinozaki T, Iwami E, et al. A case of allergic bronchopulmonary aspergillosis successfully treated with mepolizumab. BMC Pulm Med 2018; 18(1):53.

82. Oda N, Miyahara N, Senoo S, et al. Severe asthma concomitant with allergic bronchopulmonary aspergillosis successfully treated with mepolizumab. Allergol Int 2018;67(4):521–3.

83. Soeda S, To M, Kono Y, et al. Case series of allergic bronchopulmonary aspergillosis treated successfully and safely with long-term mepolizumab. Allergol Int 2019;68(3):377–9.

84. Hirota S, Kobayashi Y, Ishiguro T, et al. Allergic bronchopulmonary aspergillosis successfully treated with mepolizumab: Case report and review of the literature. Respir Med Case Rep 2019;26:59–62.

85. Altman MC, Lenington J, Bronson S, et al. Combination omalizumab and mepolizumab therapy for refractory allergic bronchopulmonary aspergillosis. J Allergy Clin Immunol Pract 2017;5(4):1137–9.

86. Soeda S, Kono Y, Tsuzuki R, et al. Allergic bronchopulmonary aspergillosis successfully treated with benralizumab. J Allergy Clin Immunol Pract 2019;7(5): 1633–5.

87. Tomomatsu K, Sugino Y, Okada N, et al. Rapid clearance of mepolizumab-resistant bronchial mucus plugs in allergic bronchopulmonary aspergillosis with benralizumab treatment. Allergol Int 2020;3–5. https://doi.org/10.1016/j.alit.2020.03.003.

88. Suzuki Y, Suda T. Eosinophilic pneumonia: A review of the previous literature, causes, diagnosis, and management. Allergol Int 2019;68(4):413–9.

89. To M, Kono Y, Yamawaki S, et al. A case of chronic eosinophilic pneumonia successfully treated with mepolizumab. J Allergy Clin Immunol Pract 2018;6(5): 1746–8.e1.

90. Lin RY, Santiago TP, Patel NM. Favorable response to asthma-dosed subcutaneous mepolizumab in eosinophilic pneumonia. J Asthma 2019;56(11):1193–7.

91. Brenard E, Pilette C, Dahlqvist C, et al. Real-life study of mepolizumab in idiopathic chronic eosinophilic pneumonia. Lung 2020;198(2):355–60.
92. Isomoto K, Baba T, Sekine A, et al. Promising effects of benralizumab on chronic eosinophilic pneumonia. Intern Med 2020;59(9):1195–8.
93. Shimizu Y, Kurosawa M, Sutoh Y, et al. Long-term treatment with anti-interleukin 5 antibodies in a patient with chronic eosinophilic pneumonia. J Investig Allergol Clin Immunol 2020;30(2):154–5.
94. Kaya H, Gümüş S, Uçar E, et al. Omalizumab as a steroid-sparing agent in chronic eosinophilic pneumonia. Chest 2012;142(2):513–6.
95. Domingo C, Pomares X. Can omalizumab be effective in chronic eosinophilic pneumonia? Chest 2013;143(1):274.
96. Shin YS, Jin HJ, Yoo H-S, et al. Successful treatment of chronic eosinophilic pneumonia with Anti-IgE therapy. J Korean Med Sci 2012;27(10):1261.
97. Laviña-Soriano E, Ampuero-López A, Izquierdo-Alonso JL. Response to omalizumab in a patient with chronic eosinophilic pneumonia and poor response to corticosteroids. Arch Bronconeumol 2018;54(7):393–4.
98. Menzella F, Montanari G, Patricelli G, et al. A case of chronic eosinophilic pneumonia in a patient treated with dupilumab. Ther Clin Risk Manag 2019;15:869–75.

Targeting Mast Cells with Biologics

Jonathan J. Lyons, MD[a],*, Dean D. Metcalfe, MD[b]

KEYWORDS

- Mast cell activation • Mastocytosis • Hereditary alpha tryptasemia • Monoclonal
- Immunotherapy

KEY POINTS

- Targeting mast cells and the effects of their mediators in individuals with allergic hypersensitivity disorders and reactions is a mainstay of therapy.
- Biologics for the treatment of allergic hypersensitivity and mast cell–associated disorders are emerging as promising second-line interventions.
- There is lack of, and a critical need for, prospective randomized blinded placebo-controlled trials of biologics in disorders where mast cells are central to the pathologic condition.
- Cytoreductive biologics, particularly those targeting neoplastic mast cells, should be reserved for select patients with aggressive and/or pernicious clonal diseases.

INTRODUCTION

Mast cells are bone marrow–derived tissue-resident cells of the myeloid lineage.[1] They reside in large numbers adjacent to blood vessels and near mucosal surfaces where they participate in aspects of both innate and adaptive immune responses and are thought to contribute to the maintenance of connective tissues and potentially other physiologic processes.[2] Mature mast cells harbor abundant secretory granules containing several biologically active preformed mediators that include proteases and histamine, which, along with lipid-derived mediators, are critical to the development of the signs and symptoms of immediate hypersensitivity reactions.[3] Release and generation of such mediators occur during highly regulated degranulation events, resulting canonically from antigen-specific immunoglobulin E (IgE) cross-linking of the

Funding: This research was supported by the Division of Intramural Research of the National Institute of Allergy and Infectious Diseases, NIH.
[a] Translational Allergic Immunopathology Unit, Laboratory of Allergic Diseases, National Institutes of Health, 9000 Rockville Pike, Building 29B, Room 5NN18, MSC 1889, Bethesda, MD 20892, USA; [b] Mast Cell Biology Section, Laboratory of Allergic Diseases, National Institute of Allergy and Infectious Diseases, National Institutes of Health, BG 10 RM 11N244B, 10 Center Drive, Bethesda, MD 20814, USA
* Corresponding author.
E-mail address: jonathan.lyons@nih.gov

high-affinity IgE bearing surface receptor FcεRI following exposure to cognate antigen.[4] However, mast cell degranulation may be thought of as a threshold event whereby several potentially additive or even synergistic pathways, including but not limited to cytokine signaling, as well as sensation of temperature, vibration, and stress signals may all contribute.[5,6] Furthermore, mast cells may be activated by cytokines and innate immune pathways to produce inflammatory cytokines independent of degranulation.[2] Many biologics have been developed, or are under development, that target mast cells directly or indirectly through inhibition of cytokines that act upon these cells and/or cytokines and other mediators produced by mast cells. In this review, the authors discuss current and future biologics that may be used to target mast cell disorders and reactions.

ROLE OF MAST CELLS IN ALLERGIC DISEASES AND REACTIONS

Mast cells are thought to be the principal mediators of acute symptoms in type I IgE-mediated immediate hypersensitivity reactions, although blood basophils may also contribute.[7] To accomplish this, mast cells both generate and release several inflammatory mediators, including but not limited to histamine, platelet-activating factor, prostaglandins, leukotrienes, and proteases, such as chymotrypsin and tryptase, the latter of which are stabilized by serglycin-bound heparin and stored within secretory granules.[1–3,7] Mast cells activated following IgE cross-linking by allergen degranulate and release these mediators, leading to vascular leak and pruritus. In addition to their role in the acute phase of allergic hypersensitivity, following activation, mast cells also contribute to the recruitment of other inflammatory cells through the production of chemokines, cytokines, and lipid mediators[8] including the recruitment and activation of eosinophils, which promotes chronic type 2 inflammation.[9] In this way, mast cells are thought to contribute not only to immediate hypersensitivity but also to several chronic allergic diatheses, including eosinophilic gastrointestinal disease (EGID), atopic dermatitis (AD), and food allergy.

CLONAL AND NONCLONAL MAST CELL–ASSOCIATED DISORDERS

In rare instances, mast cells may undergo clonal expansion, most commonly because of the acquired gain-of-function *KIT* p.D816V missense variant,[10,11] which results in constitutive activation and STAT5 phosphorylation independent of ligation by stem cell factor (SCF).[12,13] The net effect of this variant on mast cell homeostasis is at least 2-fold. First, mutant mast cells display indolent, but unrestrained growth, and second, activation of KIT-dependent pathways promotes mast cell reactivity. Together, these result in the clinical entity known as mastocytosis, which may exist in systemic or cutaneous forms as defined through established clinical criteria.[1] Individuals with mastocytosis frequently display recurrent symptoms, such as flushing, pruritus, and systemic anaphylaxis because of episodic mast cell degranulation that may occur following antigen exposure (eg, hymenoptera envenomation) or for unidentified reasons.[14,15] Indeed, individuals with systemic mastocytosis are several times more likely to experience systemic anaphylaxis than individuals in the general population.[15–19] For reasons that are less clear, urticaria and angioedema, symptoms frequently associated with mast cell mediator release, are not common clinical findings among mastocytosis patients.[20]

Symptoms observed in individuals with mastocytosis and associated with mast cell mediator release may not be limited to individuals with identifiable mast cells clones. Idiopathic anaphylaxis (IA) is an extreme example of a mast cell–associated disorder, where affected individuals experience recurrent, often severe, systemic anaphylaxis in the absence of an identifiable antigenic exposure[21]; some of these individuals may have evidence of clonal disease, but meet only 1 or 2 minor diagnostic criteria or no criteria for the clinical diagnosis of mastocytosis.[22–24] Another example is chronic spontaneous urticaria (CsU), where, as the name suggests, affected individuals have ongoing daily hives of at least 6 weeks' duration without specific provocation.[25] There are also individuals that report recurrent symptoms frequently associated with mast cell mediator release, including, but not limited to, cutaneous flushing, pruritus and/or angioedema, gastrointestinal pain, abdominal distension, vomiting and/or diarrhea, and impairment in energy and/or cognition. Many of these individuals are given the evolving diagnosis of mast cell activation syndrome (MCAS).[23,24] Although criteria for this diagnosis continue to be debated within the medical community, consensus opinion currently generally requires one of 3 clinically measurable mast cell mediators-urine arachidonic acid or histamine metabolites, or serum tryptase- be elevated during an acute symptomatic episode relative to the patient's baseline level, in order to achieve the diagnosis of MCAS.[26–28]

Finally, there are a growing number of heritable genetic conditions that lead to increased mast cell reactivity that thus far have most commonly manifested as physical urticarias.[29,30] One Mendelian genetic trait that bears mention in this context is hereditary alpha tryptasemia (HαT) caused by increased *TPSAB1* copy number encoding alpha-tryptase.[31] It is estimated that this trait may affect up to 5% of the US population and is a common cause for elevated serum tryptase, which can confound the diagnosis of MCAS.[32] Furthermore, up to two-thirds of individuals with this trait have been reported with phenotypes suggestive of mast cell mediator release, and recent mechanistic studies have demonstrated that unique enzymatic properties of alpha-tryptase containing heterotetrameric tryptases may contribute to this association.[33,34]

ALLERGEN IMMUNOTHERAPY: THE FIRST MAST CELL TARGETING BIOLOGIC

Strictly defined, biologics are treatments that are the products of living organisms or contain living organisms within them. Thus, allergen immunotherapy is the first example of the use of a biologic to target mast cell reactivity.

Paul Ehrlich first described mast cells (Mastzelle) in his doctoral dissertation in Leipzig in 1878.[35] It was not for another 30 years that the first pioneering trial in allergen immunotherapy was undertaken by Noon and Freeman,[36,37] and nearly another 50 years before the first double-blind, placebo-controlled trial was conducted demonstrating efficacy of allergen immunotherapy.[38] It was around this time, in the late 1940s and early 1950s, that mast cells were also firmly established as the culprit for immediate hypersensitivity symptoms[39,40] caused by allergens and mediated by the transferable "reaginic" substance in blood described decades earlier by Prausnitz and Kustner,[41] and later shown by Ishizaka to be γE antibodies,[42] now known as IgE. Since this pioneering work studying hay fever, there have been a large number of prospective studies using not only environmental allergens but also stinging insect extracts for individuals with venom allergy, and food antigens, administered via several routes, including subcutaneous, oral, sublingual, transdermal, and even intralymphatic.[43–45] Collectively these studies have provided strong evidence that allergen immunotherapy is safe and effective in inducing sustained nonresponsiveness to environmental and stinging insect antigens and in increasing the tolerated mass of food antigen ingestion by food allergic individuals.[44,46] Safety and efficacy of allergen immunotherapy appears to remain largely true among individuals with mast cell–associated disorders. Indeed, a prospective trial in venom allergic patients with indolent systemic mastocytosis (ISM) demonstrated venom immunotherapy (VIT) as safe and effective.[47]

However, the durability of VIT in patients with clonal disease may be diminished, and retrospective data suggest that these patients may require life-long VIT maintenance for protection from anaphylaxis resulting from field stings.[48,49]

BIOLOGICS TARGETING MAST CELL PROLIFERATION AND EFFECTOR FUNCTION
Immunoglobulin E and Allergen-Specific Monoclonal Antibodies

Much in the same way that antigen has been used to suppress mast cell reactivity, so have monoclonal antibodies been developed targeting this pathway (**Fig. 1, Table 1**). The first such biologic developed and used clinically was omalizumab, which targets IgE. Omalizumab is a humanized monoclonal IgG1 that binds to the Cε3 region of IgE, preventing association with both high- and low-affinity IgE receptors on mast cells and other cells bearing these receptors.[50] It was first Food and Drug Administration (FDA) approved for the treatment of allergic asthma in 2003.[51] Through additional mechanistic studies it was recognized that in addition to limiting immediate hypersensitivity reactions via sequestration of antigen-specific IgE, omalizumab also led to downregulation of FcεRI and suppression of mast cell reactivity.[52,53] Based in part on these findings, a trial was undertaken to examine the efficacy of omalizumab among individuals with treatment-refractory CsU.[54] Omalizumab provided significant benefit, and in 2014 received an FDA indication for this disorder. Several additional prospective studies have since demonstrated efficacy of omalizumab as an adjunctive therapy for oral and subcutaneous immunotherapy,[55–57] and still others are ongoing (NCT03881696).

Based upon these successes and the proof-of-concept that omalizumab can promote mast cell quiescence, omalizumab is frequently used in patients with mast cell–associated disorders in clinical practice. Although a relatively large number of case reports, series, and retrospective cohort studies have been largely positive on the use of omalizumab in mast cell–associated disorders,[21,58,59] including in ISM,

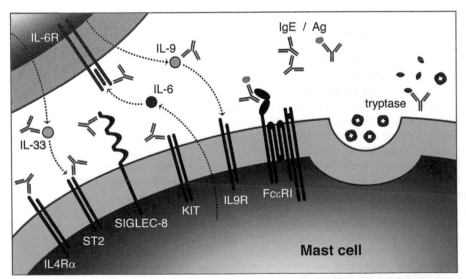

Fig. 1. Biologics targeting mast cell proliferation and effector function. Monoclonal antibodies (*red*) currently FDA approved or in phase 2/3 clinical trials that can target mast cell activation, proliferation, and/or effector functions.

Table 1		
Current and future monoclonal antibodies targeting mast cell signaling and mediators		
Target	FDA-Indication (I)/Disease Population Under Study (S)	Biologic
KIT	(S) KIT$^+$ solid tumors	CDX-0158 (formerly KTN0158)
IgE	(I) Allergic asthma, (I) CsU; (S) IA, (S) OIT	Omalizumab, ligelizumab
Allergens	(S) Allergic rhinoconjunctivitis	REGN1908-1909 (Fel d 1); REGN5713-5714-5715 (Bet v 1)
SIGLEC-8	(S) EGID, (S) allergic kerato/conjunctivitis, (S) urticarias, (S) ISM	Antolimab (AK002)
IL4Rα	(I) AD, (I) asthma, (I) CRSwNP; (S) EGID	Dupilumab
IL6R	(I) RA, (I) SJIA, (I) PJIA, (I) GCA, (I) CRS; (S) ISM[a]	Tocilizumab, sarilumab
IL-9	(F) Asthma	Enokizumab (MEDI-528)
IL-33	(S) Food allergy, (S) AD, (S) asthma, (S) CRSwNP	Etokimab (ANB-020), REGN3500, MEDI 3506
ST2	(S) Asthma,	MSTT1041A, GSK3772847
Tryptase	(S) Asthma ± allergic fungal airway disease, (S) AD, (S) COPD	MTPS9579A

Abbreviations: CRS, cytokine release syndrome; GCA, giant cell arteritis; OIT, oral immunotherapy; PJIA, polyarticular juvenile idiopathic arthritis; RA, rheumatoid arthritis; SJIA, systemic juvenile idiopathic arthritis.

[a] There are a large number of studies underway in other rheumatologic conditions using anti-IL6R.

MCAS, and IA, as well as in HαT,[60] to date only 1 randomized double-blind placebo-controlled trial in patients with IA has been undertaken to objectively examine efficacy in any of these populations (NCT00890162). The complete results are not yet published; although preliminary reported data suggest a positive effect, the study was underpowered to achieve its primary endpoint in part owing to the rigorous nature of the inclusion criteria limiting recruitment. While the preponderance of the literature would suggest that in a manner similar to that seen in patients with CsU, omalizumab has efficacy in some patients with mast cell-associated diseases, the trials to demonstrate a broader use have yet to be undertaken, and which endotypes may most benefit from this biologic remain speculative.

A second anti-IgE drug, ligelizumab, which is a humanized IgG that functions in a manner very similar to omalizumab, recently demonstrated efficacy in patients with CsU based on standardized validated symptom scores in a phase 2b study[61] and is currently in 2 phase 3 studies for CsU (NCT03907878, NCT03580356). Interestingly, in the phase 2b study, ligelizumab was reported to have greater efficacy compared with omalizumab in improving symptom scores and resolving patients' hives. However, baseline weight and total IgE were not stratified for or taken into account post hoc, and thus it is not clear whether this difference is due to a failure to meet the 0.016 mg/kg/IgE (IU/mL) therapeutic threshold for omalizumab, or if the observed increase in efficacy will be reproduced in larger ongoing trials.

Like omalizumab, the binding site of ligelizumab is in the Cε3 region of IgE, which is inaccessible once IgE is bound to FcεRI,[62] thus preventing unwanted cross-linking of receptor-bound IgE that would result in signaling and mast cell degranulation. Despite this design, between 0.09% and 0.2% of individuals who receive omalizumab develop systemic anaphylaxis,[63] typically on the first few administrations, and thus omalizumab has a black box warning associated with this risk. The mechanism underlying these rare reactions is unclear. Several hypotheses have been proposed, including non-IgE–mediated hypersensitivity to polysorbate,[64,65] an excipient contained in omalizumab preparations, and the presence of preexisting antibodies directed against some portion of omalizumab,[66] although neither has been definitely demonstrated to be the culprit. Because of this uncertainty, it is recommended that all individuals receiving this medication be observed by a medical group capable of treating anaphylaxis for 2 hours on the first 3 injections, and for 30 minutes with each subsequent injection.[66]

Recently, an alternative strategy to allergen immunotherapy has been developed whereby neutralizing monoclonal antibodies targeting major allergen components have been developed to limit immediate hypersensitivity reactions resulting from exposure. Two such targets have biologics in development. Two pooled monoclonal IgG4[P] antibodies (REGN1908 and REGN1909)- the modified isotype nomenclature indicating the presence of IgG1 sequence at the hinge-region rendering the monoclonal antibody more stable- targeting the major cat allergen Fel d 1, have completed a phase 1 study.[67] In this study, a single injection of both of the 2 noncompetitive monoclonal inhibitors given to cat-allergic individuals resulted in significant improvement in total nasal symptom scores (TNSS) following nasal provocation. Both TNSS and wheal size in response to skin-prick testing to cat hair extract was reduced for up to 85 days after injection. The mechanism underlying the potential durability of this intervention is unclear.

Using a similar strategy, another pool of 3 noncompetitive monoclonal antibodies targeting the major birch allergen Bet v 1 (REGN5713, REGN 5714, REGN5715) is currently under investigation in a 2-part phase 1 randomized, double-blind, placebo-controlled study (NCT03969849) with the same primary endpoints at the Fel d 1 study: evaluating safety and tolerability in part 1, and assessing TNSS and skin prick testing (SPT) responses to birch in part 2.

Stem Cell Factor Receptor KIT

The development of mast cell precursors in the bone marrow as well as the maintenance of long-lived mature mast cells in tissue is dependent on SCF signaling via its cognate tyrosine kinase receptor KIT. Because gain-of-function variants in KIT as well as exogenous administration of SCF to humans promote mast cell activation,[68,69] targeting this pathway to limit symptoms of immediate hypersensitivity has long been of interest. Complicating this strategy is the fact that SCF is also crucial for normal hematopoietic stem cell maturation.[70] Thus, identifying ways to inhibit this pathway while limiting marrow suppression and toxicity has been of paramount importance.

Although several small molecules have been developed to inhibit tyrosine kinase activity generally, including imatinib, nilotinib, dasatinib, midostaurin, masitinib, ibrutinib, and avapritinib, few have been KIT-specific, and most have had significant and limiting toxicity.[71] One KIT-specific biologic CDX-0158 (formerly KTN0158), a humanized monoclonal antibody that has inhibitory activity against both wild-type and mutant KIT, completed a phase 1 trial for KIT-positive advanced solid tumors in mid-2019 (NCT02642016). Although these first-in-human data are not yet available, in preclinical studies CDX-0158 reduced mast cell degranulation, mast cell number in tissues, and mast cell tumor size in canines.[72] In dogs, this monoclonal antibody resulted in anemia in 1 animal, suggesting marrow suppression may occur.

An additional intriguing strategy for targeting this pathway has been described by Garcia and colleagues.[73] They have engineered an SCF-analogue with partial agonistic activity that preferentially activates hematopoietic progenitors and does not promote mast cell activation in vitro or in mouse models. Whether such a partial agonist could be developed and applied to mast cell–associated disorders in humans remains to be seen.

Sialic Acid–Binding Immunoglobulin-Type Lectin-8

Sialic acid–binding immunoglobulin-type lectins (SIGLECs) are a family of immunoglobulin-like carbohydrate-binding molecules present primarily on the plasma membrane of immune cells that recognize specific sialic acid residues.[74] Each of the 15 known human SIGLECs display different tissue distributions and serve diverse functions. Although these molecules may contribute to cellular signaling, adhesion, and phagocytosis, most contain an intracytoplasmic domain bearing one or more immunoreceptor tyrosine-based inhibitory motif (ITIM) motifs and serve to limit immune cell activation. SIGLEC-8 was first cloned from a human with idiopathic hypereosinophilic syndrome[75] and is known to be expressed only on human allergic effector mast cells and eosinophils, and to a lesser extent on basophils.[76] Engagement of SIGLEC-8 by the endogenous ligand 6'sulfo-sialyl-Lewis-X induces eosinophil apoptosis and inhibits IgE-mediated mast cell calcium flux and degranulation.[77,78] Thus, an agonist or suicide immunoglobulin that could direct antibody-dependent cell-mediated cytotoxicity (ADCC) of allergic effector cells could be an effective treatment for mast cell–associated disorders.

Antolimab (formerly AK002) is a nonfucosylated IgG1 monoclonal antibody targeting SIGLEC-8 under study for several clinical indications. This molecule is currently given as an infusion, and owing to the lack of fucosylation, induces ADCC of blood eosinophils. In humanized mouse models, it limits systemic anaphylaxis as well as eosinophilic inflammation of the gut.[79] Ostensibly it is this ADCC activity that results in first infusion reactions, which have been described in unpublished reports of early phase studies; extension phase studies are ongoing (NCT03664960). This drug is currently being evaluated in several ongoing or recently completed clinical trials, including EGID (NCT03496571, NCT03664960), treatment-refractory urticarias, including CsU, cholinergic urticaria, and symptomatic dermatographism (NCT03436797), and a phase 1b study of severe allergic conjunctivitis (atopic keratoconjunctivitis, vernal keratoconjunctivitis, and perennial allergic conjunctivitis refractory to topical treatments) (NCT03379311). Finally, an open-label phase 1 dose-finding study in patients with ISM was also recently completed (NCT02808793). Although the preliminary data reported in these studies have thus far been positive, the results currently remain unpublished.

Cytokine and Cytokine-Receptor Blockade

In addition to the effects of SCF on mast cell reactivity and homeostasis, there are many biologics available or in development targeting other cytokines that contribute to the pathogenesis of type I hypersensitivity reactions.

Interleukin-4 (IL-4) is an early and potent driver of Th2 immune responses, contributing to skin barrier dysfunction and promoting IgE class-switching in humans.[80,81] IL-4 shares a coreceptor IL4Rα, with IL-13, which has been shown to be important for generation of high-affinity IgE associated with strong mast cell activation and severe allergic reactions in mice,[82,83] and is an important effector cytokine in allergic inflammatory responses. Both of these cytokines are generated by activated mast cells, and IL4Rα is present on the cell surface.[84–86] IL4Rα has also been shown to contribute to IL-33–associated histamine release in mouse models.[87]

Dupilumab is a fully human IgG4 monoclonal antibody that blocks receptor activation by IL-4 or IL-13. It is FDA approved for the treatment of individuals older than 12 years of age with moderate to severe AD or moderate to severe asthma, and in adults with chronic rhinosinusitis with nasal polyposis chronic rhinosinusitis with nasal polyps (CRSwNP) refractory to standard-of-care interventions.[88–90] Although it is thought that some of the efficacy observed in these atopic disorders may result from reduced activity of mast cell–derived IL-4 and IL-13 as well as reduced IL4Rα--signaling in mast cells, the mast cell–specific contribution to the pathogenesis or improvement of these diseases remains undefined in humans.

IL-6 has been demonstrated to increase proliferation and IgE-dependent activation of cultured human mast cells in vitro.[91] Individuals with ISM have been shown to have elevated levels of serum IL-6, which may contribute to several clinical symptoms, including mast cell reactivity.[92–95] Heightened serum levels in these individuals are associated with the presence of the *KIT* p.D816V gain-of-function missense variant, which promotes constitutive overexpression of IL-6 in vitro.[95] There are 2 currently FDA-approved IL-6 receptor inhibitors: tocilizumab, a humanized monoclonal IgG1, and sarilumab, a fully human monoclonal IgG1, both of which are approved for the treatment of autoimmune disease. Tocilizumab also has an indication for the treatment of cytokine release syndrome associated with chimeric antigen receptor T-cell therapy, which is thought to be a result of exuberant cytokine release from activated macrophages. Although mast cells have been implicated in the pathogenesis of joint destruction in disorders such as rheumatoid arthritis,[96] it is generally thought that other immune cells are principal drivers of autoimmune inflammation. However, the observed effects of IL-6 on the mast cell compartment among patients with ISM have led to an investigator-initiated phase 2 double-blind placebo-controlled trial of sarilumab in patients with this disorder (NCT03770273). Results are not yet available, but primary outcome measures include safety and quality of life as measured by a validated questionnaire.

IL-9 is a pleiotropic cytokine produced by several immune cell lineages, including many lymphocytes as well as mast cells.[97] Among the identified activities of this cytokine, it has been demonstrated that IL-9 can promote mast cell proliferation in vitro,[98] contributes to tissue recruitment of mast cells to sites of allergic inflammation in vitro,[99] and IL-9 produced both by mucosal mast cell and tissue homing/infiltrating Th2 cells may promote allergic phenotypes, such as AD and food allergy. Enokizumab (formerly MEDI-528) is a humanized IgG1 targeting IL-9. Despite the associations between allergic inflammation, mast cells, and IL-9, it failed in a phase 2b study of adults with uncontrolled asthma whereby no difference was seen in the Asthma Control Questionnaire-6 score, forced expiratory volume in 1 second (FEV1), or rate of exacerbation.[100]

IL-33 is a member of the IL-1 superfamily of cytokines and is expressed predominantly by cells of ectodermal and myeloid origin, including epithelia and mast cells.[101] This cytokine is produced following epithelial damage or stress and contributes to allergic inflammation via signaling through its cognate receptor ST2 found on mast cells, eosinophils, ILC2s, and Th2 lymphocytes. In this context, mast cells both produce and respond to IL-33. Etokimab (ANB020) is a humanized IgG1 anti-IL-33 monoclonal antibody that has been evaluated in phase 2a trials for AD and food allergy.[102] In the AD study, all subjects received a placebo infusion followed 1 week later by a single infusion of study drug. AD severity significantly improved as measured by a reduction in Eczema Area and Severity Index core, with maximal improvement occurring between day 29 and 57. This improvement appeared to persist in some individuals out to 150 days after infusion. Although the mast cell compartment was not evaluated in this study, another similarly sized placebo-controlled phase 2a study examined the efficacy of etokimab in peanut allergic adults.[103] In this study, 11/15 peanut-allergic individuals who received a single infusion of drug and failed an oral food challenge (OFC) at baseline were able to pass OFC at day 15, and 4 remained tolerant at day 45 after infusion. None of those receiving placebo were able to pass OFC. Despite this clinical result, there was no detectable difference in SPT responses to peanut during the study. In vivo and in vitro data suggest that short-term exposure to IL-33 can increase both IgE-dependent and -independent mast cell activation,[104,105] potentially without clear provocation in a manner dependent on IL4Rα-mediated signaling.[87]

Taken together, these results thus suggest that IL-33 blockade may be a viable therapy for prevention of mast cell activation generally, and there are several clinical trials recently completed or underway evaluating the effect of IL-33/ST2 blockade on several allergic and pulmonary diseases where mast cells may contribute. A phase 2 study of etokimab in patients with severe eosinophilic asthma (NCT03469934) was recently completed, and another in patients with CRSwNP is still recruiting (NCT03614923). Phase 2 studies of another fully human IgG4[P] anti-IL-33 monoclonal antibody REGN3500 (formerly SAR440340) in patients with AD (NCT03112577) and allergic asthma (NCT02999711) alone, or in combination with dupilumab, have recently been completed, and a third phase 2 study in chronic obstructive pulmonary disease (COPD) (NCT03546907) has also completed recruitment. A third anti-IL-33 monoclonal antibody MEDI 3506 is also recruiting adults with moderate to severe AD for a phase 2 safety and efficacy study (NCT04212169).

Within the same pathway, GSK3772847 (formerly CNTO 7160), a human IgG2 anti-ST2 monoclonal antibody, has completed a phase 2 study designed to determine efficacy in adults with moderate to severe asthma (NCT03207243) and has completed recruitment in another phase 2 study of individuals with moderate to severe asthma with concomitant allergic fungal airway disease (NCT03393806). A second anti-ST2 candidate, MSTT1041A (formerly AMG 282 and RG6149), a defucosylated fully human monoclonal antibody, has completed phase 1 study in patients with allergic asthma (NCT01928368) and CRSwNP (NCT02170337); phase 2 studies in moderate to severe AD (NCT03747575), severe asthma (NCT02918019), and COPD (NCT03615040) have also either recently been completed or have finished recruiting. Published results from all of these trials are not yet available.

Tryptase Neutralization

Although targeting mast cell mediators using antihistamines, leukotriene antagonists, and mast cell stabilizers is the mainstay of treatment of individuals with mast cell disorders, there is currently no FDA-approved biologic other than immunotherapy with allergen that targets these inflammatory molecules. However, there is renewed interest in targeting tryptase to treat allergic diseases. Human tryptases are a family of serine proteases that have only recently evolved and share only modest homology with orthologs, even those present in nonhuman primates.[106] There are 5 known tryptase loci, with TPSAB1 and TPSB2 encoding the known common secreted forms α- and/or β-tryptase.[107] Enzymatically active tryptases exist as tetrameric complexes stabilized in mast cell granules by heparin.[108] In a humanized mouse model, neutralization of enzymatically active human tryptase has been shown to reduce the severity of IgE-dependent systemic anaphylaxis.[109] Furthermore, post hoc analysis reexamining the treatment benefits of omalizumab in patients with allergic asthma suggests that a greater number of the enzymatically active β-tryptase isoform is associated with a failure to respond to this IgE-directed therapy. Based on these observations, a phase 2a, randomized, placebo-controlled, double-blind, multicenter, 2-arm study is underway to evaluate the safety and efficacy of a humanized antitryptase IgG4 monoclonal antibody (MTPS9579A) as an add-on therapy in patients with uncontrolled moderate to severe asthma (NCT04092582). The primary composite endpoint is the time to first asthma exacerbation or diary worsening. Several additional objective clinical and laboratory measures will be evaluated as secondary endpoints. Although clinical efficacy data are not yet available, targeting tryptase in mast cell–associated disorders may be of benefit as mature tryptases- in particular heterotetrameric αβ-tryptase- may contribute to many clinical phenotypes reported.[33]

BIOLOGICS TARGETING NEOPLASTIC MAST CELLS

In addition to targeting dysregulated physiologic processes that lead to enhanced mast cell activation, proliferation, or reactivity, several additional targets have been identified on neoplastic mast cells that can be targeted to eliminate mast cells (**Fig. 2**). Generally, these biologics are cytotoxic, either bearing a conjugated poisonous payload to cells they target or exhibiting strong ADCC activity (**Table 2**). Thus, these agents carry significant off-target effects and should be reserved for individuals with advanced disease or those with associated hematologic malignancies and given by physicians experienced in the care of such patients.

CD25

IL-2 is an essential cytokine for immune function.[110] Failure of IL-2 signaling, principally in T lymphocytes, because of autosomal or X-linked recessive loss-of-function mutations in one of the 3 heterotrimeric IL-2R subunits, results in combined or severe combined immunodeficiency.[111–114] IL-2 is also important for maintenance of immune tolerance, and impairment in signaling has been shown to result in loss of peripheral and self-tolerance in humans. *IL2RA* encodes the alpha subunit, which is also commonly known as CD25, which is aberrantly expressed on the surface of neoplastic mast cells,[115] where it is able to bind IL-2, but unable to signal because of the absence of IL-2Rβ. Daclizumab is an anti-CD25 humanized IgG1 monoclonal antibody approved for adults with relapsing forms of multiple sclerosis.[116] In 1 small case series, 4 patients with refractory aggressive systemic mastocytosis were treated open and off-label with daclizumab. Only 1 individual demonstrated evidence of a temporary partial clinical response with improvement in pleural effusions, ascites, flushing, emesis, diarrhea, fatigue, and joint pain over the weeks following administration of daclizumab. At that time, changes were also observed on bone marrow section, which suggested mast cell destruction. However, disease fully recurred within 1 month, and none of the other 3 individuals demonstrated benefit.[117] This drug has since been

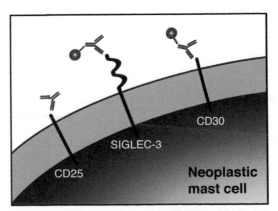

Fig. 2. FDA-approved biologics that can target neoplastic mast cells. Monoclonal antibodies (*red*) FDA approved for malignancy or immunosuppression that have shown some efficacy in case reports of patients with advanced or aggressive clonal mast cell disease.

Target	Indication	Normal Tissue Distribution	Biologic

Table 2
Food and Drug Administration–approved monoclonal antibodies that can target neoplastic mast cells

Target	Indication	Normal Tissue Distribution	Biologic
CD25	Allograft rejection prophylaxis; multiple sclerosis	Lymphocytes and activated granulocytes	Basiliximab, daclizumab[a]
CD30	Hodgkin or anaplastic lymphoma; CD30+ T-cell lymphomas	Lymphocytes and granulocytes	Brentuximab vedotin
SIGLEC-3 (CD33)	AML	Myeloid lineage cells and precursors; activated T lymphocytes	Gemtuzumab ozogamicin

[a] Voluntarily withdrawn by the manufacturer over safety concerns.

voluntarily withdrawn from the market over safety concerns.[118] Basiliximab is a chimeric IgG1 monoclonal antibody that also targets CD25 and is indicated for the acute organ rejection prophylaxis following renal transplantation.[119] This biologic has not been studied in mast cell diseases.

CD30

Tumor necrosis factor receptor superfamily member 8, or CD30, is normally expressed on the cell surface of activated T, B, and NK lymphocytes, and at a lower level in some myeloid cells, such as activated monocytes and eosinophils.[120] Ligation of CD30 by CD30L leads to NF-κB activation that can promote cellular proliferation or death. Brentuximab vedotin is a chimeric IgG1 monoclonal antibody targeting CD30 conjugated to monomethyl auristatin E (vedotin) that disrupts microtubule formation. It has several clinical indications, including advanced and high-risk Hodgkin lymphomas, systemic or cutaneous anaplastic large cell lymphoma, or other CD30-expressing peripheral T-cell lymphomas.[121] Treatment of CD30-positive systemic mastocytosis in 1 case series involving 4 patients with aggressive systemic mastocytosis (ASM) or ISM was associated with evidence of reduced disease burden in 2 patients.[122] One individual experienced partial remission with resolution of pancytopenia such that growth factor support was no longer necessary, and the patient was continued for 44 monthly cycles of drug.

Sialic Acid–Binding Immunoglobulin-Type Lectin-3 (CD33)

SIGLEC-3, or CD33, belongs to the same family of sialic acid–binding lectins as SIGLEC-8, the promising therapeutic target present on nonneoplastic mast cells.[74] In healthy individuals, CD33 is found on the surface of many myeloid lineage cells, including mast cells, as well as on activated T lymphocytes, where it serves as an inhibitory receptor regulating signaling. Gemtuzumab ozogamicin is a humanized IgG4 monoclonal antibody against CD33 that has been conjugated to a cytotoxic agent (N-acetyl gamma calicheamicin dimethyl hydrazide) approved for the treatment of CD33-positive acute myeloid leukemia (AML) in adults and reserved for relapsed or refractory CD33-positive AML in children.[123] In 1 case report, an individual with mast cell leukemia refractory to several agents, including imatinib, cladribine, and midostaurin, was treated with gemtuzumab ozogamicin resulting in complete histologic remission out to 7 months of follow-up.[124]

DISCUSSION

The utilization of biologics, in the form of allergen-specific immunotherapy, to target mast cells and their mediators in order to treat and even prevent immediate hypersensitivity symptoms and reactions has been part of clinical practice for over a century. Recent advances in technologies have massively expanded the number of monoclonal antibodies that may be used in a similar manner. Although published randomized prospective blinded placebo-controlled trials evaluating efficacy of the expanding number of biologics are generally lacking, many of these molecules hold significant promise for mast cell–associated diseases and reactions.

SUMMARY

Several biologics exist that hold promise for mast cell–associated diseases. However, only allergen immunotherapy, IgE-blocking monoclonal antibodies, and more recently, anti-IL33, have been shown to be effective in clinical trials involving clinical phenotypes resulting from mast cell activation, namely, IgE-mediated immediate hypersensitivity or CsU. Although additional studies have been completed and published results should be forthcoming, the only prospective studies of biologics in mast cell–associated disorders in the literature currently are trials of anti-IgE monoclonal therapies for CsU and VIT in ISM. Thus, prospective randomized placebo-controlled clinical trials of biologics in mast cell–associated diseases are critically needed because efficacy in CsU or other allergic diseases, such as asthma and AD, may not translate to the mast cell compartment.

CLINICAL CARE POINTS

- Diagnostic criteria for MCAS are incompletely defined and unevenly applied by physicians, making the care and study of individuals with this diagnosis very challenging.
- VIT is safe and effective but potentially less durable in patients with ISM who may require lifelong maintenance to ensure protection from field stings.
- Anti-IgE therapy is effective for antihistamine-refractory CsU, but case reports and cohort studies suggest it may not effectively treat many other symptoms frequently attributed to mast cell activation.
- There are no prospective studies to support off-label use of any monoclonal antibody in clonal or non-clonal mast cell–associated diseases.
- Cytoreductive biologics should be reserved for patients with aggressive clonal mast cell disease and administered only by physicians experienced in caring for these complex patients.

DISCLOSURE

The authors declare no competing or conflicting interests.

REFERENCES

1. Metcalfe DD. Mast cells and mastocytosis. Blood 2008;112(4):946–56.
2. Olivera A, Beaven MA, Metcalfe DD. Mast cells signal their importance in health and disease. J Allergy Clin Immunol 2018;142(2):381–93.
3. Wernersson S, Pejler G. Mast cell secretory granules: armed for battle. Nat Rev Immunol 2014;14(7):478–94.

4. Turner H, Kinet JP. Signalling through the high-affinity IgE receptor Fc epsilonRI. Nature 1999;402(6760 Suppl):B24–30.

5. Halova I, Ronnberg E, Draberova L, et al. Changing the threshold-signals and mechanisms of mast cell priming. Immunol Rev 2018;282(1):73–86.

6. Gilfillan AM, Peavy RD, Metcalfe DD. Amplification mechanisms for the enhancement of antigen-mediated mast cell activation. Immunol Res 2009; 43(1–3):15–24.

7. Galli SJ, Tsai M. IgE and mast cells in allergic disease. Nat Med 2012;18(5): 693–704.

8. Theoharides TC, Alysandratos KD, Angelidou A, et al. Mast cells and inflammation. Biochim Biophys Acta 2012;1822(1):21–33.

9. Shakoory B, Fitzgerald SM, Lee SA, et al. The role of human mast cell-derived cytokines in eosinophil biology. J Interferon Cytokine Res 2004;24(5):271–81.

10. Longley BJ, Tyrrell L, Lu SZ, et al. Somatic c-KIT activating mutation in urticaria pigmentosa and aggressive mastocytosis: establishment of clonality in a human mast cell neoplasm. Nat Genet 1996;12(3):312–4.

11. Nagata H, Worobec AS, Oh CK, et al. Identification of a point mutation in the catalytic domain of the protooncogene c-kit in peripheral blood mononuclear cells of patients who have mastocytosis with an associated hematologic disorder. Proc Natl Acad Sci U S A 1995;92(23):10560–4.

12. Furitsu T, Tsujimura T, Tono T, et al. Identification of mutations in the coding sequence of the proto-oncogene c-kit in a human mast cell leukemia cell line causing ligand-independent activation of c-kit product. J Clin Invest 1993; 92(4):1736–44.

13. Baumgartner C, Cerny-Reiterer S, Sonneck K, et al. Expression of activated STAT5 in neoplastic mast cells in systemic mastocytosis: subcellular distribution and role of the transforming oncoprotein KIT D816V. Am J Pathol 2009;175(6): 2416–29.

14. Kors JW, van Doormaal JJ, de Monchy JG. Anaphylactoid shock following Hymenoptera sting as a presenting symptom of systemic mastocytosis. J Intern Med 1993;233(3):255–8.

15. Bonadonna P, Zanotti R, Muller U. Mastocytosis and insect venom allergy. Curr Opin Allergy Clin Immunol 2010;10(4):347–53.

16. Gulen T, Hagglund H, Dahlen B, et al. High prevalence of anaphylaxis in patients with systemic mastocytosis - a single-centre experience. Clin Exp Allergy 2014;44(1):121–9.

17. Brockow K, Jofer C, Behrendt H, et al. Anaphylaxis in patients with mastocytosis: a study on history, clinical features and risk factors in 120 patients. Allergy 2008;63(2):226–32.

18. Sheikh A, Hippisley-Cox J, Newton J, et al. Trends in national incidence, lifetime prevalence and adrenaline prescribing for anaphylaxis in England. J R Soc Med 2008;101(3):139–43.

19. Wood RA, Camargo CA Jr, Lieberman P, et al. Anaphylaxis in America: the prevalence and characteristics of anaphylaxis in the United States. J Allergy Clin Immunol 2014;133(2):461–7.

20. Alvarez-Twose I, Gonzalez de Olano D, Sanchez-Munoz L, et al. Clinical, biological, and molecular characteristics of clonal mast cell disorders presenting with systemic mast cell activation symptoms. J Allergy Clin Immunol 2010;125(6): 1269–78.e2.

21. Carter MC, Akin C, Castells MC, et al. Idiopathic anaphylaxis yardstick: practical recommendations for clinical practice. Ann Allergy Asthma Immunol 2020; 124(1):16–27.

22. Valent P, Akin C, Metcalfe DD, et al. 2016 updated WHO classification and novel emerging treatment concepts. Blood 2017;129(11):1420–7.

23. Akin C. Mast cell activation syndromes. J Allergy Clin Immunol 2017;140(2): 349–55.

24. Picard M, Giavina-Bianchi P, Mezzano V, et al. Expanding spectrum of mast cell activation disorders: monoclonal and idiopathic mast cell activation syndromes. Clin Ther 2013;35(5):548–62.

25. Saini SS. Chronic spontaneous urticaria: etiology and pathogenesis. Immunol Allergy Clin North Am 2014;34(1):33–52.

26. Akin C, Valent P, Metcalfe DD. Mast cell activation syndrome: proposed diagnostic criteria. J Allergy Clin Immunol 2010;126(6):1099–104.e4.

27. Valent P, Akin C, Arock M, et al. Definitions, criteria and global classification of mast cell disorders with special reference to mast cell activation syndromes: a consensus proposal. Int Arch Allergy Immunol 2012;157(3):215–25.

28. Valent P, Akin C, Bonadonna P, et al. Proposed diagnostic algorithm for patients with suspected mast cell activation syndrome. J Allergy Clin Immunol Pract 2019;7(4):1125–33.e1.

29. Ombrello MJ, Remmers EF, Sun G, et al. Cold urticaria, immunodeficiency, and autoimmunity related to PLCG2 deletions. N Engl J Med 2012;366(4):330–8.

30. Boyden SE, Desai A, Cruse G, et al. Vibratory urticaria associated with a missense variant in ADGRE2. N Engl J Med 2016;374(7):656–63.

31. Lyons JJ, Yu X, Hughes JD, et al. Elevated basal serum tryptase identifies a multisystem disorder associated with increased TPSAB1 copy number. Nat Genet 2016;48(12):1564–9.

32. Lyons JJ. Hereditary alpha tryptasemia: genotyping and associated clinical features. Immunol Allergy Clin North Am 2018;38(3):483–95.

33. Le QT, Lyons JJ, Naranjo AN, et al. Impact of naturally forming human alpha/beta-tryptase heterotetramers in the pathogenesis of hereditary alpha-tryptasemia. J Exp Med 2019;216(10):2348–61.

34. Lyons JJ, Chovanec J, O'Connell MP, et al. Heritable risk for severe anaphylaxis associated with increased α-tryptase-encoding germline copy number at TPSAB1. J Allergy Clin Immunol 2020.

35. Beiträge PE. Zur Theorie und Praxis der histologischen Färbung [doctoral thesis]. Germany: University of Leipzig; 1878. Available at: https://www.worldcat.org/title/beitrage-fur-theorie-und-praxis-der-histologischen-farbung/oclc/63372150.

36. Prophylactic LN. Innoculation against hay fever. Lancet 1911;177(4580):2. Available at: https://www.thelancet.com/journals/lancet/article/PIIS0140-6736(00)78276-6/fulltext.

37. Freeman J. Further observations on the treatment of hay fever by hypodermic inoculations of pollen vaccine. Lancet 1911;178(4594):4.

38. Frankland AW, Augustin R. Prophylaxis of summer hay-fever and asthma: a controlled trial comparing crude grass-pollen extracts with the isolated main protein component. Lancet 1954;266(6821):1055–7.

39. Rocha e Silva M, Scroggie AE, Fidlar E, et al. Liberation of histamine and heparin by peptone from the isolated dog's liver. Proc Soc Exp Biol Med 1947;64(2): 141–6.

40. Riley JF, West GB. Histamine in tissue mast cells. J Physiol 1952;117(4):72P–3P.

41. Prausnitz CKH. Studien über die Überempfindlichkeit. Centralbl Bakterio 1921; 86:160.
42. Ishizaka K, Ishizaka T. Identification of gamma-E-antibodies as a carrier of reaginic activity. J Immunol 1967;99(6):1187–98.
43. Gunawardana NC, Durham SR. New approaches to allergen immunotherapy. Ann Allergy Asthma Immunol 2018;121(3):293–305.
44. Wood RA. Food allergen immunotherapy: current status and prospects for the future. J Allergy Clin Immunol 2016;137(4):973–82.
45. Golden DB. Insect sting allergy and venom immunotherapy: a model and a mystery. J Allergy Clin Immunol 2005;115(3):439–47 [quiz: 48].
46. Akdis CA, Akdis M. Mechanisms of allergen-specific immunotherapy and immune tolerance to allergens. World Allergy Organ J 2015;8(1):17.
47. Bonadonna P, Gonzalez-de-Olano D, Zanotti R, et al. Venom immunotherapy in patients with clonal mast cell disorders: efficacy, safety, and practical considerations. J Allergy Clin Immunol Pract 2013;1(5):474–8.
48. Bonadonna P, Zanotti R, Pagani M, et al. Anaphylactic reactions after discontinuation of hymenoptera venom immunotherapy: a clonal mast cell disorder should be suspected. J Allergy Clin Immunol Pract 2018;6(4):1368–72.
49. Oude Elberink JN, de Monchy JG, Kors JW, et al. Fatal anaphylaxis after a yellow jacket sting, despite venom immunotherapy, in two patients with mastocytosis. J Allergy Clin Immunol 1997;99(1 Pt 1):153–4.
50. Pennington LF, Tarchevskaya S, Brigger D, et al. Structural basis of omalizumab therapy and omalizumab-mediated IgE exchange. Nat Commun 2016;7:11610.
51. Busse WW. Anti-immunoglobulin E (omalizumab) therapy in allergic asthma. Am J Respir Crit Care Med 2001;164(8 Pt 2):S12–7.
52. Gomez G, Jogie-Brahim S, Shima M, et al. Omalizumab reverses the phenotypic and functional effects of IgE-enhanced Fc epsilonRI on human skin mast cells. J Immunol 2007;179(2):1353–61.
53. Beck LA, Marcotte GV, MacGlashan D, et al. Omalizumab-induced reductions in mast cell Fce psilon RI expression and function. J Allergy Clin Immunol 2004; 114(3):527–30.
54. Maurer M, Rosen K, Hsieh HJ, et al. Omalizumab for the treatment of chronic idiopathic or spontaneous urticaria. N Engl J Med 2013;368(10):924–35.
55. Brandstrom J, Vetander M, Sundqvist AC, et al. Individually dosed omalizumab facilitates peanut oral immunotherapy in peanut allergic adolescents. Clin Exp Allergy 2019;49(10):1328–41.
56. Takahashi M, Soejima K, Taniuchi S, et al. Oral immunotherapy combined with omalizumab for high-risk cow's milk allergy: a randomized controlled trial. Sci Rep 2017;7(1):17453.
57. Yee CSK, Albuhairi S, Noh E, et al. Long-term outcome of peanut oral immunotherapy facilitated initially by omalizumab. J Allergy Clin Immunol Pract 2019; 7(2):451–61.e7.
58. Broesby-Olsen S, Vestergaard H, Mortz CG, et al. Omalizumab prevents anaphylaxis and improves symptoms in systemic mastocytosis: efficacy and safety observations. Allergy 2018;73(1):230–8.
59. Lemal R, Fouquet G, Terriou L, et al. Omalizumab therapy for mast cell-mediator symptoms in patients with ISM, CM, MMAS, and MCAS. J Allergy Clin Immunol Pract 2019;7(7):2387–95.e3.
60. Mendoza Alvarez LB, Barker R, Nelson C, et al. Clinical response to omalizumab in patients with hereditary alpha-tryptasemia. Ann Allergy Asthma Immunol 2020;124(1):99–100.e1.

61. Maurer M, Gimenez-Arnau AM, Sussman G, et al. Ligelizumab for chronic spontaneous urticaria. N Engl J Med 2019;381(14):1321–32.

62. Gasser P, Tarchevskaya SS, Guntern P, et al. The mechanistic and functional profile of the therapeutic anti-IgE antibody ligelizumab differs from omalizumab. Nat Commun 2020;11(1):165.

63. Lieberman PL, Jones I, Rajwanshi R, et al. Anaphylaxis associated with omalizumab administration: risk factors and patient characteristics. J Allergy Clin Immunol 2017;140(6):1734–6.e4.

64. Lieberman P. The unusual suspects: a surprise regarding reactions to omalizumab. Allergy Asthma Proc 2007;28(3):259–61.

65. Perino E, Freymond N, Devouassoux G, et al. Xolair-induced recurrent anaphylaxis through sensitization to the excipient polysorbate. Ann Allergy Asthma Immunol 2018;120(6):664–6.

66. Cox L, Platts-Mills TA, Finegold I, et al. American Academy of Allergy, Asthma & Immunology/American College of Allergy, Asthma and Immunology Joint Task Force Report on omalizumab-associated anaphylaxis. J Allergy Clin Immunol 2007;120(6):1373–7.

67. Orengo JM, Radin AR, Kamat V, et al. Treating cat allergy with monoclonal IgG antibodies that bind allergen and prevent IgE engagement. Nat Commun 2018; 9(1):1421.

68. Costa JJ, Demetri GD, Harrist TJ, et al. Recombinant human stem cell factor (kit ligand) promotes human mast cell and melanocyte hyperplasia and functional activation in vivo. J Exp Med 1996;183(6):2681–6.

69. Moskowitz CH, Stiff P, Gordon MS, et al. Recombinant methionyl human stem cell factor and filgrastim for peripheral blood progenitor cell mobilization and transplantation in non-Hodgkin's lymphoma patients–results of a phase I/II trial. Blood 1997;89(9):3136–47.

70. Broudy VC. Stem cell factor and hematopoiesis. Blood 1997;90(4):1345–64.

71. Bibi S, Arock M. Tyrosine kinase inhibition in mastocytosis: KIT and beyond KIT. Immunol Allergy Clin North Am 2018;38(3):527–43.

72. London CA, Gardner HL, Rippy S, et al. KTN0158, a humanized anti-KIT monoclonal antibody, demonstrates biologic activity against both normal and malignant canine mast cells. Clin Cancer Res 2017;23(10):2565–74.

73. Ho CCM, Chhabra A, Starkl P, et al. Decoupling the functional pleiotropy of stem cell factor by tuning c-Kit signaling. Cell 2017;168(6):1041–1052 e18.

74. Macauley MS, Crocker PR, Paulson JC. Siglec-mediated regulation of immune cell function in disease. Nat Rev Immunol 2014;14(10):653–66.

75. Kikly KK, Bochner BS, Freeman SD, et al. Identification of SAF-2, a novel siglec expressed on eosinophils, mast cells, and basophils. J Allergy Clin Immunol 2000;105(6 Pt 1):1093–100.

76. Kiwamoto T, Kawasaki N, Paulson JC, et al. Siglec-8 as a drugable target to treat eosinophil and mast cell-associated conditions. Pharmacol Ther 2012;135(3): 327–36.

77. Nutku E, Aizawa H, Hudson SA, et al. Ligation of Siglec-8: a selective mechanism for induction of human eosinophil apoptosis. Blood 2003;101(12):5014–20.

78. Yokoi H, Choi OH, Hubbard W, et al. Inhibition of FcepsilonRI-dependent mediator release and calcium flux from human mast cells by sialic acid-binding immunoglobulin-like lectin 8 engagement. J Allergy Clin Immunol 2008;121(2): 499–505.e1.

79. Youngblood BA, Brock EC, Leung J, et al. Siglec-8 antibody reduces eosinophils and mast cells in a transgenic mouse model of eosinophilic gastroenteritis. JCI Insight 2019;4(19):e126219.
80. Paul WE. History of interleukin-4. Cytokine 2015;75(1):3–7.
81. Sehra S, Yao Y, Howell MD, et al. IL-4 regulates skin homeostasis and the predisposition toward allergic skin inflammation. J Immunol 2010;184(6):3186–90.
82. Fallon PG, Emson CL, Smith P, et al. IL-13 overexpression predisposes to anaphylaxis following antigen sensitization. J Immunol 2001;166(4):2712–6.
83. Gowthaman U, Chen JS, Zhang B, et al. Identification of a T follicular helper cell subset that drives anaphylactic IgE. Science 2019;365(6456):eaaw6433.
84. Burton OT, Darling AR, Zhou JS, et al. Direct effects of IL-4 on mast cells drive their intestinal expansion and increase susceptibility to anaphylaxis in a murine model of food allergy. Mucosal Immunol 2013;6(4):740–50.
85. McLeod JJ, Baker B, Ryan JJ. Mast cell production and response to IL-4 and IL-13. Cytokine 2015;75(1):57–61.
86. Toru H, Pawankar R, Ra C, et al. Human mast cells produce IL-13 by high-affinity IgE receptor cross-linking: enhanced IL-13 production by IL-4-primed human mast cells. J Allergy Clin Immunol 1998;102(3):491–502.
87. Komai-Koma M, Brombacher F, Pushparaj PN, et al. Interleukin-33 amplifies IgE synthesis and triggers mast cell degranulation via interleukin-4 in naive mice. Allergy 2012;67(9):1118–26.
88. Bachert C, Han JK, Desrosiers M, et al. Efficacy and safety of dupilumab in patients with severe chronic rhinosinusitis with nasal polyps (LIBERTY NP SINUS-24 and LIBERTY NP SINUS-52): results from two multicentre, randomised, double-blind, placebo-controlled, parallel-group phase 3 trials. Lancet 2019; 394(10209):1638–50.
89. Castro M, Corren J, Pavord ID, et al. Dupilumab efficacy and safety in moderate-to-severe uncontrolled asthma. N Engl J Med 2018;378(26):2486–96.
90. Simpson EL, Bieber T, Guttman-Yassky E, et al. Two phase 3 trials of dupilumab versus placebo in atopic dermatitis. N Engl J Med 2016;375(24):2335–48.
91. Desai A, Jung MY, Olivera A, et al. IL-6 promotes an increase in human mast cell numbers and reactivity through suppression of suppressor of cytokine signaling 3. J Allergy Clin Immunol 2016;137(6):1863–71.e6.
92. Brockow K, Akin C, Huber M, et al. IL-6 levels predict disease variant and extent of organ involvement in patients with mastocytosis. Clin Immunol 2005;115(2): 216–23.
93. Mayado A, Teodosio C, Garcia-Montero AC, et al. Increased IL6 plasma levels in indolent systemic mastocytosis patients are associated with high risk of disease progression. Leukemia 2016;30(1):124–30.
94. Theoharides TC, Boucher W, Spear K. Serum interleukin-6 reflects disease severity and osteoporosis in mastocytosis patients. Int Arch Allergy Immunol 2002;128(4):344–50.
95. Tobio A, Bandara G, Morris DA, et al. Oncogenic D816V-KIT signaling in mast cells causes persistent IL-6 production. Haematologica 2020;105(1):124–35.
96. Shin K, Nigrovic PA, Crish J, et al. Mast cells contribute to autoimmune inflammatory arthritis via their tryptase/heparin complexes. J Immunol 2009;182(1): 647–56.
97. Goswami R, Kaplan MH. A brief history of IL-9. J Immunol 2011;186(6):3283–8.
98. Hultner L, Druez C, Moeller J, et al. Mast cell growth-enhancing activity (MEA) is structurally related and functionally identical to the novel mouse T cell growth factor P40/TCGFIII (interleukin 9). Eur J Immunol 1990;20(6):1413–6.

99. Sehra S, Yao W, Nguyen ET, et al. TH9 cells are required for tissue mast cell accumulation during allergic inflammation. J Allergy Clin Immunol 2015; 136(2):433–40.e1.

100. Oh CK, Leigh R, McLaurin KK, et al. A randomized, controlled trial to evaluate the effect of an anti-interleukin-9 monoclonal antibody in adults with uncontrolled asthma. Respir Res 2013;14:93.

101. Liew FY, Girard JP, Turnquist HR. Interleukin-33 in health and disease. Nat Rev Immunol 2016;16(11):676–89.

102. Chen YL, Gutowska-Owsiak D, Hardman CS, et al. Proof-of-concept clinical trial of etokimab shows a key role for IL-33 in atopic dermatitis pathogenesis. Sci Transl Med 2019;11(515):eaax2945.

103. Chinthrajah S, Cao S, Liu C, et al. Phase 2a randomized, placebo-controlled study of anti-IL-33 in peanut allergy. JCI Insight 2019;4(22):e131347.

104. Joulia R, L'Faqihi FE, Valitutti S, et al. IL-33 fine tunes mast cell degranulation and chemokine production at the single-cell level. J Allergy Clin Immunol 2017;140(2):497–509 e10.

105. Wang Z, Guhl S, Franke K, et al. IL-33 and MRGPRX2-triggered activation of human skin mast cells-elimination of receptor expression on chronic exposure, but reinforced degranulation on acute priming. Cells 2019;8(4):341.

106. Trivedi NN, Tong Q, Raman K, et al. Mast cell alpha and beta tryptases changed rapidly during primate speciation and evolved from gamma-like transmembrane peptidases in ancestral vertebrates. J Immunol 2007;179(9):6072–9.

107. Caughey GH. Tryptase genetics and anaphylaxis. J Allergy Clin Immunol 2006; 117(6):1411–4.

108. Schwartz LB, Lewis RA, Austen KF. Tryptase from human pulmonary mast cells. Purification and characterization. J Biol Chem 1981;256(22):11939–43.

109. Maun HR, Jackman JK, Choy DF, et al. An allosteric anti-tryptase antibody for the treatment of mast cell-mediated severe asthma. Cell 2019;179(2): 417–31.e19.

110. Malek TR. The biology of interleukin-2. Annu Rev Immunol 2008;26:453–79.

111. Fernandez IZ, Baxter RM, Garcia-Perez JE, et al. A novel human IL2RB mutation results in T and NK cell-driven immune dysregulation. J Exp Med 2019;216(6): 1255–67.

112. Schmalstieg FC, Leonard WJ, Noguchi M, et al. Missense mutation in exon 7 of the common gamma chain gene causes a moderate form of X-linked combined immunodeficiency. J Clin Invest 1995;95(3):1169–73.

113. Sharfe N, Dadi HK, Shahar M, et al. Human immune disorder arising from mutation of the alpha chain of the interleukin-2 receptor. Proc Natl Acad Sci U S A 1997;94(7):3168–71.

114. Zhang Z, Gothe F, Pennamen P, et al. Human interleukin-2 receptor beta mutations associated with defects in immunity and peripheral tolerance. J Exp Med 2019;216(6):1311–27.

115. Sotlar K, Horny HP, Simonitsch I, et al. CD25 indicates the neoplastic phenotype of mast cells: a novel immunohistochemical marker for the diagnosis of systemic mastocytosis (SM) in routinely processed bone marrow biopsy specimens. Am J Surg Pathol 2004;28(10):1319–25.

116. Baldassari LE, Rose JW. Daclizumab: development, clinical trials, and practical aspects of use in multiple sclerosis. Neurotherapeutics 2017;14(4):842–58.

117. Quintas-Cardama A, Amin HM, Kantarjian H, et al. Treatment of aggressive systemic mastocytosis with daclizumab. Leuk Lymphoma 2010;51(3):540–2.

118. The L. End of the road for daclizumab in multiple sclerosis. Lancet 2018; 391(10125):1000.
119. Salis P, Caccamo C, Verzaro R, et al. The role of basiliximab in the evolving renal transplantation immunosuppression protocol. Biologics 2008;2(2):175–88.
120. van der Weyden CA, Pileri SA, Feldman AL, et al. Understanding CD30 biology and therapeutic targeting: a historical perspective providing insight into future directions. Blood Cancer J 2017;7(9):e603.
121. Donato EM, Fernandez-Zarzoso M, Hueso JA, et al. Brentuximab vedotin in Hodgkin lymphoma and anaplastic large-cell lymphoma: an evidence-based review. Onco Targets Ther 2018;11:4583–90.
122. Borate U, Mehta A, Reddy V, et al. Treatment of CD30-positive systemic mastocytosis with brentuximab vedotin. Leuk Res 2016;44:25–31.
123. Laszlo GS, Estey EH, Walter RB. The past and future of CD33 as therapeutic target in acute myeloid leukemia. Blood Rev 2014;28(4):143–53.
124. Alvarez-Twose I, Martinez-Barranco P, Gotlib J, et al. Complete response to gemtuzumab ozogamicin in a patient with refractory mast cell leukemia. Leukemia 2016;30(8):1753–6.

Biologics and Allergy Immunotherapy in the Treatment of Allergic Diseases

Linda Cox, MD

KEYWORDS

- Allergy immunotherapy • Subcutaneous immunotherapy
- Sublingual immunotherapy • Rhinosinusitis with nasal polyps • Atopic dermatitis
- Biologics • Omalizumab • Mepolizumab

KEY POINTS

- Effective, safe, and inexpensive therapies for chronic allergic conditions remain a significant unmet need.
- Allergy immunotherapy through the sublingual and subcutaneous route has demonstrated clinical and cost efficacy in the treatment of allergic rhinitis and asthma, but adherence with both routes is problematic.
- Several biologics targeting specific components of the immune system have demonstrated efficacy in patient populations not responding to conventional medical treatment.
- Anti-immunoglobulin E therapy, omalizumab, has been shown to be effective in moderate to severe asthmatics not well controlled on inhaled corticosteroids and long-acting beta agonist, chronic urticaria, and allergic rhinitis.
- Agents targeting interleukin 5 (IL-5), mepolizumab, benralizumab, reslizumab have demonstrated efficacy and poorly controlled asthmatics with eosinophilic phenotype.
- Dupilumab, an agent targeting IL-4/IL-13 has been shown to be effective in moderate to severe atopic dermatitis and allergic asthma. In patients with severe chronic rhinosinusitis with polys, dupilumab reduced polyp size, sinus opacification, and symptom severity.

INTRODUCTION

Allergic diseases, which include asthma, allergic rhinitis, chronic rhinosinusitis, atopic dermatitis, and food allergies, represent some of most common chronic pediatric and adult conditions worldwide. The 3 most common allergic diseases, asthma, allergic rhinitis, and atopic dermatitis often present during childhood and continue to be symptomatic through adulthood if they are not adequately managed. Medical management may include avoidance of known allergenic and nonallergenic triggers, pharmacotherapy, and immunomodulatory therapies. Ideally, complete avoidance of the

1108 South Wolcott Street, Casper, WY 82601, USA
E-mail address: lscoxmd@gmail.com

Immunol Allergy Clin N Am 40 (2020) 687–700
https://doi.org/10.1016/j.iac.2020.06.008
0889-8561/20/© 2020 Elsevier Inc. All rights reserved.

offending allergen would be the optimal management approach, but this is rarely achievable. In addition, there are limited data indicating any single environmental control measure will result in improved outcomes. A Cochrane systematic review of randomized controlled trials that compared the effectiveness of several bedroom environmental control measures in dust mite (HDM) perennial allergic rhinitis found that isolated use of HDM impermeable bedding did not seem to be effective.[1] Similarly, there is little evidence indicating cat/dog removal from the household will improve allergic rhinitis or asthma symptoms.[2] This "failure to improve" after cat/dog removal may be due to the persistence of airborne animal dander long after removal[3] or the ubiquitous presence of animal dander.[4] It may be difficult to predict and avoid exposure to irritant triggers, such as fragrance/chemical odors and cold air. Pharmacotherapy is aimed at controlling symptoms and preventing exacerbations. Most allergy medications need to be administered one or more times a day even during asymptomatic periods. Adherence is as problematic as with any chronic condition.[5] One study found that only 25% of asthmatic children were compliant with prescribed regimens.[5] Concerns about medication adverse effects, costs, side-effects, and absence of active symptoms are likely contributing factors to the high rate of medication nonadherence in allergic conditions. These factors should be considered along with the risks and benefits of long-term therapy during the medical management decision-making process. Immunomodulators that target specific components of the immune system are another therapeutic option in the management of allergic disease. Compared with conventional pharmacotherapy, they offer the advantage of less frequent administration and potentially less adverse effects. The purpose of this paper is to review the efficacy and safety of biologics in the treatment of allergic rhinitis, chronic rhinosinusitis, asthma, and atopic dermatitis.

Allergy Immunotherapy

The oldest biological therapy for allergic disease that is still in current use is allergy immunotherapy (AIT). It entails administration of the identified allergen at repeated intervals over a 3- to 5-year period. The frequency of administration will vary with administration route. The treatment specific for the aeroallergen is identified during the allergy diagnostic evaluation. The allergen extracts are derived from natural sources (pollen) or cultures (mold/fungi and house dust mite). Influenced by the success of Jenner's work with the smallpox vaccine, physicians in the early 1900s theorized that they could induce a similar immunity by injecting "hay fever" patients with pollen extracts. Initial experiments were hampered with high rate of systemic allergic reactions.[6] The first successful report of subcutaneous immunotherapy (SCIT) against "hay fever" was reported by Noon in a 1911 Lancet article.[7] Patients were administered incrementally higher doses of a pollen extract, which Noon had prepared by extracting pollen in distilled water and freeze-thawing and boiling. Conjunctival allergen provocation test was used to confirm allergy sensitivity and monitor response to allergy immunotherapy. Noon noted that efficacy and safety were related allergen dose, which he summarized in the following statement: "an overdose can induce a severe attack of hay fever lasting 24 hours" and "sensibility of hay fever patients may be decreased by properly directed dosage."[7] Since Noon's report, numerous studies confirmed the safety and efficacy of SCIT in the treatment of allergic rhinitis and asthma.

However, it was not until many decades later that the mechanisms responsible for its efficacy began to be elucidated. AIT induces several immunologic changes that likely contribute to the sustained immune-specific tolerance associated with effective AIT. These include changes in allergen-specific T- and B-cell cytokine responses, increase in allergen-specific immunoglobulin G4 (IgG4), production of antibodies capable of blocking allergen presentation, and reductions in mast cell, eosinophil, and basophil activation.[8] The immunologic changes take place at different time points in the AIT course. Mast cell and basophil desensitization occurs early in the treatment course followed by induction of the generation of T and B regulatory cells producing IL-10 and other cytokines, which result in suppression of effector TH_1 and TH_2 cells.[8] AIT is considered the only proven disease-modifying treatment of allergic disease. AIT's disease-modifying effects include altering the progression of the allergic disease, for example, development of asthma or new allergen sensitizations and the induction of long-term clinical tolerance, for example, preventing insect sting anaphylaxis. In contrast to pharmacotherapy, AIT can provide symptomatic improvement that may continue for years after therapy discontinuation.[9,10]

SCIT continues to be prescribed in a manner largely unchanged from Noon's protocol of administering unmodified extracts in increasing doses over a period of weeks to months. The major disadvantage of SCIT is the relatively narrow margin between therapeutic efficacy and adverse side effects. Because of the risk of systemic allergic reactions that include rare life-threatening anaphylaxis, it is recommended that SCIT be administered in a medically supervised setting with an appropriate wait period.[11] Efforts to develop safer and more effective AIT led to investigations with modified allergens and alternate delivery routes.

Multiple randomized-controlled clinical trials demonstrated the safety and efficacy of sublingual immunotherapy, administered as a tablet or liquid extract. Although few studies have directly compared SCIT and sublingual immunotherapy treatment (SLIT), their efficacy seems comparable. However, SLIT clearly has the more favorable safety profile, which allows for home administration. Currently there are only 4 Food Drug Administration (FDA)-approved tablets in the United States (see **Table 1** for summary of approved products). In the United States, SLIT with liquid extracts is considered "off-label" treatment. "Off-label" treatment is not generally covered by third-party payers.

The recommended treatment duration for SLIT and SCIT is at least 3 years of monthly maintenance injections or daily tablet ingestion. There is little difference between the 2 routes in terms of adherence, which has been shown to be equally poor and comparable to adherence rates with long-term pharmacotherapy.[5] In 3 retrospective claims-based analysis studies, the rate of premature discontinuation of treatment was 45% to 93% of SLIT and 41% to 77% of SCIT patients.[12] Cost and inconvenience were of the most commonly cited reasons for discontinuation.[12]

The other alternative AIT routes that have demonstrated efficacy in the treatment of allergic rhinitis/rhinoconjunctivitis are epicutaneous (EPIT) and intralymphatic immunotherapy (ILIT). In EPIT, the allergen is applied to skin in the form of a patch. A double-blind, placebo-controlled (DBPC) trial of 98 grass pollen allergic rhinoconjunctivitis patients examined the efficacy of one preseasonal EPIT course on 2 subsequent pollen seasons.[13] Patients were randomized to receive 6 weekly grass pollen extract or placebo patches. The patches were applied to tape-stripped skin that remained on the skin for 8 hours 6-weekly. Allergen EPIT was associated with a median symptom improvement of 48% and 40% in the first and second treatment-free season, respectively as compared with 10% and 15% improvement after placebo ($P = .003$). Allergen EPIT was also associated with a significant decrease in conjunctival allergen reactivity and increase in allergen-specific IgG4 ($P<.001$). Adverse reactions were primarily eczema at the application site. One patient experienced a grade 2 systemic allergic reaction. EPIT also seems to be a promising treatment of food allergies.[14] The FDA had granted Viaskin Peanut Patch Fast Track and Breakthrough Therapy Designation

Table 1
Federal Drug Administration–approved sublingual immunotherapy products

	ORALAIR	RAGWITEK	GRASTEK	ODACTA
Manufacturer	Stallergens	Merck & Co	Merck & Co	Merck & Co
Indications	Grass pollen–induced allergic rhinitis with or without conjunctivitis	Short ragweed pollen–induced allergic rhinitis with or without conjunctivitis	Timothy grass pollen–induced allergic rhinitis with or without conjunctivitis	Dust mite–induced allergic rhinitis with or without conjunctivitis
Ages	10–65 y	18–65 y	5–65 y	18–65 y
Dosage	100 IR, 300 IRA Age 10–17 y: Day 1: 100 IR Day2: 2 x 100 IR Day3 and following: 300 IR Age 18–65 y Day 1 and following: 300 IR	1 tablet daily, 12 Amb a 1-unit	1 tablet daily, 2800 bioequivalent allergy units (BAUs)	12 SQ-HDM, major allergen content not provided
First dose administration	Observe patients in the office for at least 30 min following the initial dose			
Instructions for dose administration	Place the tablet under the tongue for at least 1 min, until completely dissolved, then swallow			
Active ingredients	Grass pollen mix: Sweet Vernal, Orchard, Perennial Rye, Timothy, Kentucky Blue Grass	Short ragweed pollen	Timothy grass pollen	1:1:1 potency ratio of D. farinae group 1 allergen, D. farinae group 2 allergen, D. pteronyssinus group 1 allergen, and D. pteronyssinus group 2 allergen

Inactive ingredients	Mannitol, microcrystalline cellulose, croscarmellose sodium, colloidal anhydrous silica, magnesium stearate, and lactose monohydrate			Gelatin NF (fish source)[a], mannitol USP, and sodium hydroxide NF
Initiation of therapy in relation to pollen season	Four months before the expected onset of each grass pollen season and continue throughout the season	At least 12 wk before the expected onset of ragweed pollen season and continue throughout the season	At least 12 wk before the expected onset of grass pollen season and continue throughout the season; for sustained effectiveness for one grass pollen season after cessation of treatment, GRASTEK may be taken daily for 3 consecutive years	Not specified/applicable
Contraindications	• Severe, unstable, or uncontrolled asthma • History of any severe systemic allergic reaction or any severe local reaction to SLIT • Hypersensitivity to any of the inactive ingredients contained in this product • A history of eosinophilic esophagitis			
Precautions	• Prescribe autoinjectable epinephrine, instruct and train patients on its appropriate use, and instruct patients to seek immediate medical care on its use			

[a] Gelatin is derived from a skin of cold-water fish source such as cod, pollock, or haddock. Gelatin constitutes a fraction of the 28 mg tablet weight. In one study, commercial, food-grade fish gelatin derived from the skins of codfish was evaluated in a double-blind, placebo-controlled food challenge. None of the 30 fish-allergic patients reacted adversely to the ingestion of cumulative dose of 3.61 g fish gelatin. Investigators concluded with a 95% certainty that 90% of fish-allergic consumers will not react to ingestion of a 3.61 g cumulative dose of fish gelatin.[61]

(DBV Technologies, Montrouge, France). The company submitted a Biologics License Application for Viaskin Peanut Patch for the treatment of peanut-allergic children aged 4 to 11 years to the FDA in October 2019. Questions regarding efficacy and the patch's adhesion to the skin prompted the FDA to cancel the Allergenic Products Advisory Committee meeting, which was convened to discuss approval for patch's approval.[15]

ILIT offers the advantage of a short treatment course that seems to have an efficacy similar to SCIT and SLIT. An open trial, ILIT with 3 injections of grass pollen administered at 4-week intervals resulted in significant improvement in nasal allergen challenge after 4 months and symptomatic improvement comparable to 3 years of SCIT.[16] Subsequent DBPC ILIT trials have reported conflicting results. One DBPC trial of 36 patients with allergic rhinoconjunctivitis reported a significant improvement in seasonal allergy symptom with ILIT.[17] Another DBPC trial of 45 patients with grass-pollen allergic rhinoconjunctivitis reported no improvement in clinical or immunologic parameters with ILIT.[18] Another consideration with ILIT is that if may be difficult to locate inguinal lymph nodes in obese individuals.

At present, ILIT and EPIT are considered investigational and SCIT and SLIT are the only routes recommended in practice guidelines for the treatment of allergic rhinitis, asthma, and some cases of atopic dermatitis.[11,19–21] Although, asthma is an indication for AIT, there have been no studies of SLIT or SCIT in poorly controlled severe asthma. In addition, "severe asthma uncontrolled by pharmacotherapy" is considered a relative contraindication for SCIT and SLIT.[11,22]

TARGETED BIOLOGICAL THERAPIES
Omalizumab

Until the development of biologics targeting specific components of the immune system, management of severe asthma generally required multiple medications, that is, inhaled corticosteroids, long-acting beta-agonist, prednisone, etc. AIT is generally not an option because poorly controlled asthma has been identified as a risk factor for severe and fatal AIT reactions.[23] Management challenges related to polypharmacy adherence, suboptimal control despite adherence, and long -term medication adverse effects, for example, prednisone, prompted investigations of biological agents directed at specific components of the allergic inflammatory pathway.

The first biological agent for the treatment of moderate to severe asthma, omalizumab (Xolair; Genentech), was approved in the United States in 2003. It is a 95% humanized monoclonal antibody directed against the Fc portion of IgE. Omalizumab binds the Cε3 domain of the Fc, which prevents IgE binding to the high-affinity IgE receptor FcεR1 and subsequent effector cell activation.[24] Significant and rapid reductions in free serum IgE has been demonstrated after one dose of omalizumab.[25] In one study, mean serum IgE levels were decreased by 96% three days after omalizumab administration.[26] As serum IgE levels decreases, there is a reduction in the expression FcεR1 receptor on multiple cell types, for example, mast cells, basophils, dendritic cells, etc.[26,27] In the study cited earlier, omalizumab treatment was also associated with a 73% reduction in basophil FcεR1 receptor expression within 7 days and a 90% reduction in basophil responsiveness at 90 days. In multiple clinical trials, omalizumab treatment resulted in reduced inhaled corticosteroid (ICS) dose and beta-agonist rescue inhaler use, fewer asthma exacerbations, and improved asthma symptoms.[24] Omalizumab has been shown to decrease the frequency of fall seasonal asthma exacerbations in adolescents and children.[28,29] The major cause of fall seasonal asthma exacerbations is viral respiratory tract infections such as, rhinovirus. In a randomized-controlled trial comparing omalizumab add-on treatment with guidelines-based asthma care, there was a reduced duration and frequency of rhinovirus infections in the omalizumab-treated group.[30] In another DBPC study, omalizumab resulted in a greater interferon-alpha responses to rhinovirus and fewer asthma exacerbations.[28] These studies provide evidence that omalizumab may decrease susceptibility to rhinovirus infections and subsequent asthma exacerbations.[30] This effect has not been demonstrated with any other asthma therapeutic agent.

According to the Global Initiative for Asthma 2020 update, anti-IgE therapy should be considered as add-on therapy for adolescents, adults, and children, aged 6 to 11 years, with asthma poorly controlled on moderate dose ICS and long-acting beta-agonist (ie, step 5 treatment).[31]

Omalizumab was later FDA approved for chronic urticaria. The speculated mechanisms for omalizumab's efficacy in chronic urticaria, a nonatopic condition, include reduced mast cell sensitivity, blockage of IgG autoantibodies directed against IgE or the FcεRI receptor or blockage of IgE autoantibodies directed against an antigen to be identified.[32]

Omalizumab has also been studied in several other conditions. It was shown to be effective in reducing nasal symptom scores and improving quality of life and several studies of seasonal and perennial allergic rhinitis.[24] Despite demonstrated efficacy, omalizumab was not approved by the FDA for the treatment of allergic rhinitis. The cost of treatment may have been a factor in the FDA's decision.[33] Clinical trials investigating omalizumab as treatment of atopic dermatitis have yielded conflicting data. A recent systematic review and meta-analysis reported that only 43% of patients with atopic dermatitis responded omalizumab.[34] A series of case reports suggest omalizumab may be effective in allergic bronchopulmonary aspergillosis, systemic mastocytosis, and eosinophilic granulomatosis with polyangiitis.[24] Pretreatment with omalizumab has been shown to improve the safety of rush and cluster aeroallergen immunotherapy and oral food immunotherapy.[35–38] Omalizumab added to AIT provided an additional 48% improvement compared with AIT alone.[39]

The most common adverse reaction from omalizumab is injection-site pain and bruising. The package insert contains additional warnings regarding malignancies, geohelminth infections, cardiovascular diseases, and a "black box" warning concerning anaphylaxis. A "black box" is the most serious type of warning mandated by the US Food and Drug Administration (FDA) in pharmaceutical package inserts.[40] The warning was based on a review of spontaneous postmarketing adverse events submitted to the FDA suggesting that at least 0.2% of patients who received Xolair (omalizumab) experienced anaphylaxis.[41] The review also noted that many of the cases were delayed in onset and characterized by a protracted progression. Based on the anaphylaxis warning, a Joint Task Force of the American Academy of Allergy, Asthma and Immunology and the American College of Allergy, Asthma and Immunology (omalizumab Joint Task Force) published a report recommending omalizumab patients be prescribed an epinephrine autoinjector and be observed for 2 hours after the first 3 injections and 30 minutes for all subsequent injections.[42,43]

Initial pooled analysis of phase I and II trials reported a higher incidence of malignancies in omalizumab-treated group compared with the control group (0.5% vs 0.2%).[44] The malignancies were heterogeneous in tumor type and organ and most of the cases (60%) were diagnosed within 6 months of treatment.[45] Subsequently, multicenter, prospective, observational cohort study entitled Evaluating the Clinical Effectiveness and Long-Term Safety in Patients with Moderate to Severe Asthma found no significant difference in the adjusted malignancy rate between the omalizumab-treated (n = 5007) and nonomalizumab group (n = 2829).

Biologics Targeting Interleukin 5

Interleukin 5 (IL-5) is a TH2 cytokine that plays a key role in eosinophil activation. Since 2017, the FDA has approved 3 anti-IL-5 therapies as add-on therapy for severe asthmatics with an eosinophilic phenotype: benralizumab (Fasenra; AstraZeneca), a humanized monoclonal antibody directed against IL-5Rα; mepolizumab (Nucala; GalxoSmithKline), a neutralizing anti-IL-5 antibody; and reslizumab (Cinqair), an IgG4κ monoclonal antibody targeting circulating IL-5. The pivotal trials differed in how they defined an eosinophilic phenotype and asthma exacerbation. Mepolizumab and benralizumab trials required that patients have eosinophil counts greater that 150 cells/μL and reslizumab required that patients have an eosinophil count greater than or equal to 400 cells/μL. This has practical implications as clinical trial's inclusion criteria can influence health insurance coverage policies. Other differences between the agents include administration route, dosing frequency, and safety warnings. Mepolizumab and benralizumab are administered subcutaneously and reslizumab is administered intravenously. Reslizumab and mepolizumab are administered every 4 weeks. Benralizumab is also administered every 4 weeks for the first 3 infusions and thereafter every 8 weeks. Reslizumab has an additional "black box" safety warning regarding anaphylaxis that states "healthcare professionals should be prepared to manage anaphylaxis that can be life-threatening that and must be administered in a healthcare setting by a healthcare professional prepared to manage anaphylaxis."[46] However, the product information for reslizumab and mepolizumab indicate that it should be administered by a health care professional. A systematic review and meta-analysis of biological agents targeting eosinophilic inflammation in type 2 asthma found that all 3 anti-IL-5 associated with significant reductions in asthma exacerbation with no superiority of one biological over the others.[47] As no anti-IL-5 agent demonstrated superior clinically efficacy, it is likely that benralizumab would be a preferred agent due to its less frequent dosing requirement.

Dupilumab

Dupilumab (Dupixent; Regeneron) is a humanized monoclonal antibody directed at IL-4α, which blocks the signaling of IL-4 and IL-13, which are key cytokines involved in the differentiation of TH2 lymphocytes from naïve T cells.[48] It was initially approved in 2017 for treatment of moderate to severe atopic dermatitis. It was subsequently approved in 2018 for the treatment of moderate to severe asthma and in 2019 for the treatment of chronic rhinosinusitis with nasal polys. It is administered subcutaneously every 2 weeks. Administration can be performed at home or in the clinic setting.

Atopic dermatitis is a chronic relapsing inflammatory skin condition effecting approximately 15% to 20% of children and 1% to 3% of adults worldwide.[49] The incidence of atopic dermatitis has increased 2- to 3-fold in industrialized nations since the 1970s. Before dupilumab approval, topical corticosteroids and hydration were the mainstay of atopic dermatitis treatment and safe and effective treatment of severe atopic dermatitis was a significant unmet need. The FDA granted the application for dupilumab Priority Review and Breakthrough Therapy Designation because of this unmet need.[50]

A systematic review and meta-analysis evaluated the safety and efficacy of dupilumab for the treatment of moderate to severe atopic dermatitis and reviewed 6 randomized-controlled trials involving 2447 patients.[51] Compared with placebo, dupilumab treatment resulted in significant improvements in Eczema Area and Severity Index score (standardized mean difference [SMD] = −0.89, 95% confidence interval [CI] −1.0 to −0.78), greater reduction in percentage of body surface area affected

(SMD = −0.83, 95% CI −0.90 to −0.75), pruritus numeric rating scale scores (SMD = −0.81, 95% CI −0.96 to −0.66), and Dermatology Life Quality Index scores (SMD = −0.78, 95% CI −0.89 to −0.66). Dupilumab resulted in greater proportion of patients achieving Investigator's Global Assessment response (relative risk = 3.82; 95% CI 3.23–4.51), which was the primary outcome in the pivotal clinical trials.[51]

In a large DBPC of 1902 patients 12 years of age or older with uncontrolled asthma that compared add-on dupilumab with placebo, dupilumab resulted in 47.7% reduction in asthma exacerbations compared with placebo.[52] Dupilumab treatment was also associated with a significant increase in FEV(1) (0.32 L vs 0.14 L in matched placebo group; $P<.001$).[52]

Dupilumab was the first biological approved for the treatment of chronic rhinosinusitis with nasal polyps (CRSwNP).[53] CRSwNP is a chronic inflammatory condition associated with significant morbidity and decreased quality of life with an estimated prevalence of 4·2% in the United States and 4·3% in Europe.[54] Approximately 25% to 30% of patients with chronic rhinosinusitis have CRSwNP.[55] There are limited effective medical treatment options for CRSwNP, for example, nasal corticosteroids, nasal saline irrigation, and oral corticosteroids. Patients failing medical therapy may require sinus surgery and repeated courses of oral corticosteroids. In addition, nasal polyps may reoccur despite sinus surgery and appropriate postoperative medical management. Patients with both CRSwNP and asthma require, on average, significantly more sinus surgeries than patients with CRSwNP alone.[55]

Two multinational, multicenter, randomized DBPC parallel-group studies evaluated the efficacy of dupilumab as add-on therapy to standard of care in 728 adults with severe CRSwNP.[54] Severe CRSwNP inclusion criteria were based on symptoms, medical/surgical history, and examination findings. Included patients had to have bilateral nasal polyps, symptoms of chronic rhinosinusitis despite intranasal corticosteroid use, and a bilateral endoscopic nasal polyp score of at least 5 (maximum 8). Inclusion criteria also required a history of received systemic corticosteroids in the preceding 2 years or previous sinonasal surgery.

Dupilumab significantly improved the coprimary endpoints in both studies. At 24 weeks, least squares mean difference in NPS of dupilumab treatment versus placebo was -2·06 (95% CI -2·43 to -1·69; p<0·0001) i difference in nasal congestion or obstruction score was -0·89 (-1·07 to -0·71; p<0·0001) i; and difference in Lund-Mackay CT scores was -7·44 (-8·35 to -6·53; p<0·0001).

There were no significant safety issues in the dupilumab asthma and CRSwNP trials. However, in atopic dermatitis trials, dupilumab associated with a higher incidence of conjunctivitis (8.6%–22.1%) compared with those receiving placebo (2.1%–11.1%).[56] The pathogenesis of dupilumab-induced conjunctivitis is unknown. Management depends on the symptoms severity but should include an ophthalmology consultation for new-onset conjunctivitis. In most case, patients are able to continue dupilumab with medical management of their conjunctivitis. Dupilumab is available as a prefilled syringe or pen that can be self-administered at a dosing frequency of every 4 weeks.

SUMMARY: PRACTICAL CONSIDERATIONS AND UNMET NEEDS

One of the most significant unmet need in the management of chronic allergic diseases such as asthma, chronic rhinosinusitis, and atopic dermatitis is the availability of safe, effective, inexpensive, and convenient therapies. Ideally, such therapies would be disease modifying and potentially curative. Until this past decade, allergy immunotherapy was the only immune modifying treatment. However, for several reasons, which include convenience and safety, SCIT has only been prescribed to a small percentage of allergic patients (2%–9% in the United States).[12] SLIT offers the advantage of a better safety profile and home administration, but adherence has been shown to be equally as poor as SCIT and pharmacotherapy with other chronic conditions. In addition, neither immunotherapy route has been studied in severe allergic asthma. Biologics targeting IL-5, IgE, and IL-4/IL-13 have expanded the therapeutic options for allergic asthma and other refractory allergic conditions. Dupilumab offers the advantage of home administration and has an indication for 3 conditions: atopic dermatitis, asthma, and rhinosinusitis with nasal polys. SCIT is relatively inexpensive and has shown to significantly reduce health care costs compared with standard drug treatment.[57–59] Single-allergen SLIT has also been shown to be cost-effective, but multiallergen SLIT could be cost-prohibitive.[60] All of the biologics have substantial monetary costs, which can amount to thousands of dollars a month. Although these expenses are often covered by third-party payers, obtaining authorization approval can be challenging.

In summary, the armamentarium for chronic allergic disease management includes pharmacotherapy, SLIT, SCIT, and several biological agents targeting specific components of the immune system. There continues to be a need for less expensive and more effective therapies that could potentially lead to long-term remissions after discontinuation.

CLINICS CARE POINTS

- AIT is the only treatment of allergic asthma and allergic rhinitis with proven post-treatment clinical efficacy and favorable immunologic changes. There have been limited studies examining the optimal duration of AIT, but it seems that at least 3 years is necessary for persistent posttreatment efficacy. Studies have demonstrated that adherence with SCIT and SLIT is equally poor. Indications for AIT include allergic asthma, allergic rhinitis, atopic dermatitis, and peanut allergy.

- Omalizumab is a biological agent that targets IgE. It was initially approved for moderate to severe allergic asthma and later approved for chronic urticaria. Dosage for allergic asthma depends on IgE level and body weight. Patients with IgE levels that do not fall within the product information range (30 to 700 IU/ml for adultsadolescents 12 and older and 30-1300 IU/ml in children 6 to <12 years old) product information dosing guide would generally not. The product information includes a warning about anaphylaxis. Thus, it is recommended that omalizumab be administered in medically supervised setting.

- Three biological agents targeting IL-5 have been approved for the treatment of severe asthma with an eosinophilic phenotype: benralizumab, a humanized monoclonal antibody directed against IL-5Rα; mepolizumab, a neutralizing anti-IL-5 antibody; and reslizumab, an IgG4κ monoclonal antibody targeting circulating IL-5. There are no direct studies comparing these products but a systematic review and meta-analysis found no evidence that one product was superior to another in reducing asthma exacerbations. Product preference may depend on the administration guidelines. The products differ in their product information warnings and administration route and frequency. Benralizumab and mepolizumab are administered subcutaneously at 8- and 4-week intervals, respectively. Reslizumab is administered intravenously at 4-week intervals and has a "black-box" warning regarding anaphylaxis. The product information for all 3 indicate they should be administered by a health care provider.

- Dupilumab is a biological agent that targets IL-4/IL-13. It offers the advantage of treating 3 allergic conditions. It was initially approved for atopic dermatitis and later for allergic asthma and chronic rhinosinusitis with nasal polys. Another advantage is that it can be self-administered in the home setting.

- All of the biological agents are relatively expensive, and the treatment duration is indefinite. None to date have demonstrated persistent posttreatment efficacy. It is likely that their use will be limited to patients with more severe and difficult-to-treat allergic disease.

CONFLICT OF INTEREST

None.

REFERENCES

1. Sheikh A, Hurwitz B, Nurmatov U, et al. House dust mite avoidance measures for perennial allergic rhinitis. Cochrane Database Syst Rev 2010;(7):CD001563.
2. Portnoy JM, Kennedy K, Sublett JL, et al. Environmental assessment and exposure control: a practice parameter–furry animals. Ann Allergy Asthma Immunol 2012;108(4):223.e1.
3. Wood RA, Chapman MD, Adkinson NF Jr, et al. The effect of cat removal on allergen content in household-dust samples. J Allergy Clin Immunol 1989;83(4): 730–4.
4. Arbes SJ Jr, Cohn RD, Yin M, et al. Dog allergen (Can f 1) and cat allergen (Fel d 1) in US homes: results from the National Survey of Lead and Allergens in Housing. J Allergy Clin Immunol 2004;114(1):111–7.
5. Bender BG, Oppenheimer J. The Special Challenge of Nonadherence With Sublingual Immunotherapy. J Allergy Clin Immunol In Pract 2014;2(2):152–5.
6. Bachmann MF, Kündig TM. Allergen-specific immunotherapy: is it vaccination against toxins after all? Allergy 2017;72(1):13–23.
7. Noon L. Prophylactic inoculation against hay fever. Lancet 1911;1:1572–3.
8. Akdis M, Akdis CA. Mechanisms of allergen-specific immunotherapy: multiple suppressor factors at work in immune tolerance to allergens. J Allergy Clin Immunol 2014;133(3):621–31.
9. Durham SR, Emminger W, Kapp A, et al. SQ-standardized sublingual grass immunotherapy: confirmation of disease modification 2 years after 3 years of treatment in a randomized trial. J Allergy Clin Immunol 2012;129(3):717–25.e5.
10. Marogna M, Spadolini I, Massolo A, et al. Long-lasting effects of sublingual immunotherapy according to its duration: a 15-year prospective study. J Allergy Clin Immunol 2010;126(5):969–75.
11. Cox L, Nelson H, Lockey R, et al. Allergen immunotherapy: a practice parameter third update. J Allergy Clin Immunol 2011;127(1):S1–55.
12. Cox LS, Hankin C, Lockey R. Allergy immunotherapy adherence and delivery route: location does not matter. J Allergy Clin Immunol In Pract 2014;2(2):156–60.
13. Senti G, von Moos S, Tay F, et al. Determinants of efficacy and safety in epicutaneous allergen immunotherapy: summary of three clinical trials. Allergy 2015; 70(6):707–10.
14. Waldron J, Kim EH. Sublingual and Patch Immunotherapy for Food Allergy. Immunol Allergy Clin North Am 2020;40(1):135–48.
15. Dearment A. FDA cancels AdCom meeting for DBV's peanut allergy patch, citing efficacy concerns. MedCityNews 2020. Available at: https://medcitynews.com/2020/03/fda-cancels-adcom-meeting-for-dbvs-peanut-allergy-patch-citing-efficacy-concerns/. Accessed May 28, 2020.

16. Senti G, Prinz Vavricka BM, Erdmann I, et al. Intralymphatic allergen administration renders specific immunotherapy faster and safer: a randomized controlled trial. Proc Natl Acad Sci U S A 2008;105(46):17908–12.

17. Hylander T, Larsson O, Petersson-Westin U, et al. Intralymphatic immunotherapy of pollen-induced rhinoconjunctivitis: a double-blind placebo-controlled trial. Respir Res 2016;17(1):10.

18. Witten M, Malling HJ, Blom L, et al. Is intralymphatic immunotherapy ready for clinical use in patients with grass pollen allergy? J Allergy Clin Immunol 2013; 132(5):1248–52.e5.

19. Agache I, Lau S, Akdis CA, et al. EAACI Guidelines on Allergen Immunotherapy: House dust mite-driven allergic asthma. Allergy 2019;74(5):855–73.

20. Roberts G, Pfaar O, Akdis CA, et al. EAACI Guidelines on Allergen Immunotherapy: Allergic rhinoconjunctivitis. Allergy 2018;73(4):765–98.

21. Schneider L, Tilles S, Lio P, et al. Atopic dermatitis: a practice parameter update 2012. J Allergy Clin Immunol 2013;131(2):295–9.e1-27.

22. Greenhawt M, Oppenheimer J, Nelson M, et al. Sublingual immunotherapy: A focused allergen immunotherapy practice parameter update. Ann Allergy Asthma Immunol 2017;118(3):276–82.e2.

23. Bernstein DI, Epstein TEG. Safety of allergen immunotherapy in North America from 2008-2017: Lessons learned from the ACAAI/AAAAI National Surveillance Study of adverse reactions to allergen immunotherapy. Allergy Asthma Proc 2020;41(2):108–11.

24. Polk P, Stokes J. Anti-IgE therapy. In: Cox LS, editor. Immunotherapies for allergic disease. 1. Philadelphia: Elsevier Health Sciences; 2019. p. 355–72.

25. MacGlashan DW Jr, Bochner BS, Adelman DC, et al. Down-regulation of Fc(epsilon)RI expression on human basophils during in vivo treatment of atopic patients with anti-IgE antibody. J Immunol 1997;158(3):1438–45.

26. Lin H, Boesel KM, Griffith DT, et al. Omalizumab rapidly decreases nasal allergic response and FcÎµRI on basophils. J Allergy Clin Immunol 2004;113(2):297–302.

27. Prussin C, Griffith DT, Boesel KM, et al. Omalizumab treatment downregulates dendritic cell FcepsilonRI expression. J Allergy Clin Immunol 2003;112(6): 1147–54.

28. Teach SJ, Gill MA, Togias A, et al. Preseasonal treatment with either omalizumab or an inhaled corticosteroid boost to prevent fall asthma exacerbations. J Allergy Clin Immunol 2015;136(6):1476–85.

29. Busse WW, Morgan WJ, Gergen PJ, et al. Randomized trial of omalizumab (anti-IgE) for asthma in inner-city children. N Engl J Med 2011;364(11):1005–15.

30. Esquivel A, Busse WW, Calatroni A, et al. Effects of omalizumab on rhinovirus infections, illnesses, and exacerbations of asthma. Am J Respir Crit Care Med 2017;196(8):985–92.

31. Global initiative for asthma global strategy for maagement and prevention 2020 update. Available at: https://ginasthma.org/gina-reports. Accessed May 29, 2020.

32. Kaplan AP, Giménez-Arnau AM, Saini SS. Mechanisms of action that contribute to efficacy of omalizumab in chronic spontaneous urticaria. Allergy 2017;72(4): 519–33.

33. Vashisht P, Casale T. Omalizumab for treatment of allergic rhinitis. Expert Opin Biol Ther 2013;13(6):933–45.

34. Wang HH, Li YC, Huang YC. Efficacy of omalizumab in patients with atopic dermatitis: A systematic review and meta-analysis. J Allergy Clin Immunol 2016;138(6):1719–22.e1.

35. Casale TB, Busse WW, Kline JN, et al. Omalizumab pretreatment decreases acute reactions after rush immunotherapy for ragweed-induced seasonal allergic rhinitis. J Allergy Clin Immunol 2006;117(1):134–40.

36. Massanari M, Nelson H, Casale T, et al. Effect of pretreatment with omalizumab on the tolerability of specific immunotherapy in patients with persistent symptomatic asthma inadequately controlled with inhaled corticosteroids. Ann Allergy Asthma Immunol 2009;102(1 supplement):17.

37. Nadeau KC, Schneider LC, Hoyte L, et al. Rapid oral desensitization in combination with omalizumab therapy in patients with cow's milk allergy. J Allergy Clin Immunol 2011;127(6):1622–4.

38. Wood RA, Kim JS, Lindblad R, et al. A randomized, double-blind, placebo-controlled study of omalizumab combined with oral immunotherapy for the treatment of cow's milk allergy. J Allergy Clin Immunol 2016;137(4):1103–10.e11.

39. Kuehr J, Brauburger J, Zielen S, et al. Efficacy of combination treatment with anti-IgE plus specific immunotherapy in polysensitized children and adolescents with seasonal allergic rhinitis. J Allergy Clin Immunol 2002;109(2):274–80.

40. Aaronson D. The "black box" warning and allergy drugs. J Allergy Clin Immunol 2006;117(1):40–4.

41. Limb SL, Starke PR, Lee CE, et al. Delayed onset and protracted progression of anaphylaxis after omalizumab administration in patients with asthma. J Allergy Clin Immunol 2007;120(6):1378–81.

42. Cox L, Platts-Mills TA, Finegold I, et al. American Academy of Allergy, Asthma & Immunology/American College of Allergy, Asthma and Immunology Joint Task Force Report on omalizumab-associated anaphylaxis. J Allergy Clin Immunol 2007;120(6):1373–7.

43. Cox L, Lieberman P, Wallace D, et al. American Academy of Allergy, Asthma & Immunology/American College of Allergy, Asthma & Immunology Omalizumab-Associated Anaphylaxis Joint Task Force follow-up report. J Allergy Clin Immunol 2011;128(1):210–2.

44. Xolair® (Omalizumab) for Subcutaneous Use—Genentech, Inc.. 2008. Available at: http://www.xolair.com/prescribing_information.html.

45. Data on file. Genentech and Novartis Pharmeuticals Corporation; 2008.

46. Cinquair. Available at: https://www.cinqair.com/globalassets/cinqair/prescribing information.pdf. Accessed May 30, 2020.

47. Wang FP, Liu T, Lan Z, et al. Efficacy and safety of anti-interleukin-5 therapy in patients with asthma: a systematic review and meta-analysis. PLoS One 2016; 11(11):e0166833.

48. Rosenwasser L, Patel N. Effect of immunomodulators on allergen immunotherapy. In: Cox L, editor. Immunotherapies for allergic disease. Philadelphia: Elsevier; 2019.

49. Avena-Woods C. Overview of atopic dermatitis. Am J Manag Care 2017;23(8 Suppl):S115–23.

50. Available at: https://www.fda.gov/news-events/press-announcements/fda-approves-new-eczema-drug-dupixent. Accessed May 30, 2020.

51. Wang FP, Tang XJ, Wei CQ, et al. Dupilumab treatment in moderate-to-severe atopic dermatitis: A systematic review and meta-analysis. J Dermatol Sci 2018; 90(2):190–8.

52. Castro M, Corren J, Pavord ID, et al. Dupilumab efficacy and safety in moderate-to-severe uncontrolled asthma. N Engl J Med 2018;378(26):2486–96.

53. Franzese CB. The role of biologics in the treatment of nasal polyps. Immunol Allergy Clin North Am 2020;40(2):295–302.

54. Bachert C, Han JK, Desrosiers M, et al. Efficacy and safety of dupilumab in patients with severe chronic rhinosinusitis with nasal polyps (LIBERTY NP SINUS-24 and LIBERTY NP SINUS-52): results from two multicentre, randomised, double-blind, placebo-controlled, parallel-group phase 3 trials. Lancet 2019; 394(10209):1638–50.

55. Stevens WW, Schleimer RP, Kern RC. Chronic Rhinosinusitis with Nasal Polyps. J Allergy Clin Immunol In Pract 2016;4(4):565–72.

56. Agnihotri G, Shi K, Lio PA. A clinician's guide to the recognition and management of dupilumab-associated conjunctivitis. Drugs R D 2019;19(4):311–8.

57. Cox LS, Murphey A, Hankin C. The cost-effectiveness of allergen immunotherapy compared with pharmacotherapy for treatment of allergic rhinitis and asthma. Immunol Allergy Clin 2020;40(1):69–85.

58. Hankin CS, Cox L, Bronstone A, et al. Allergy immunotherapy: reduced health care costs in adults and children with allergic rhinitis. J Allergy Clin Immunol 2013;131(4):1084–91.

59. Meadows A, Kaambwa B, Novielli N, et al. A systematic review and economic evaluation of subcutaneous and sublingual allergen immunotherapy in adults and children with seasonal allergic rhinitis. Health Technol Assess 2013;17(27): vi, xi-xiv, 1-322.

60. Cox L. Sublingual immunotherapy for aeroallergens: status in the United States. Allergy Asthma Proc 2014;35(1):34–42.

61. Hansen TK, Poulsen LK, Stahl Skov P, et al. A randomized, double-blinded, placebo-controlled oral challenge study to evaluate the allergenicity of commercial, food-grade fish gelatin. Food and chemical toxicology : an international journal published for the British Industrial Biological Research Association 2004;42: 2037–44.

UNITED STATES POSTAL SERVICE ® Statement of Ownership, Management, and Circulation (All Periodicals Publications Except Requester Publications)

1. Publication Title	2. Publication Number	3. Filing Date
IMMUNOLOGY AND ALLERGY CLINICS OF NORTH AMERICA	006 – 361	9/18/2020

4. Issue Frequency	5. Number of Issues Published Annually	6. Annual Subscription Price
FEB, MAY, AUG, NOV	4	$344.00

7. Complete Mailing Address of Known Office of Publication (Not printer) (Street, city, county, state, and ZIP+4®)

ELSEVIER INC.
230 Park Avenue, Suite 800
New York, NY 10169

Contact Person
Malathi Samayan
Telephone (Include area code)
91-44-4299-4507

8. Complete Mailing Address of Headquarters or General Business Office of Publisher (Not printer)

ELSEVIER INC.
230 Park Avenue, Suite 800
New York, NY 10169

9. Full Names and Complete Mailing Addresses of Publisher, Editor, and Managing Editor (Do not leave blank)

Publisher (Name and complete mailing address)

Dolores Meloni, ELSEVIER INC.
1600 JOHN F KENNEDY BLVD. SUITE 1800
PHILADELPHIA, PA 19103-2899

Editor (Name and complete mailing address)

KATERINA HEIDHAUSEN, ELSEVIER INC.
1600 JOHN F KENNEDY BLVD. SUITE 1800
PHILADELPHIA, PA 19103-2899

Managing Editor (Name and complete mailing address)

PATRICK MANLEY, ELSEVIER INC.
1600 JOHN F KENNEDY BLVD. SUITE 1800
PHILADELPHIA, PA 19103-2899

10. Owner (Do not leave blank. If the publication is owned by a corporation, give the name and address of the corporation immediately followed by the names and addresses of all stockholders owning or holding 1 percent or more of the total amount of stock. If not owned by a corporation, give the names and addresses of the individual owners. If owned by a partnership or other unincorporated firm, give its name and address as well as those of each individual owner. If the publication is published by a nonprofit organization, give its name and address.)

Full Name	Complete Mailing Address
WHOLLY OWNED SUBSIDIARY OF REED/ELSEVIER, US HOLDINGS	1600 JOHN F KENNEDY BLVD. SUITE 1800 PHILADELPHIA, PA 19103-2899

11. Known Bondholders, Mortgagees, and Other Security Holders Owning or Holding 1 Percent or More of Total Amount of Bonds, Mortgages, or Other Securities. If none, check box ▶ ☐ None

Full Name	Complete Mailing Address
N/A	

12. Tax Status (For completion by nonprofit organizations authorized to mail at nonprofit rates) (Check one)
The purpose, function, and nonprofit status of this organization and the exempt status for federal income tax purposes:
☒ Has Not Changed During Preceding 12 Months
☐ Has Changed During Preceding 12 Months (Publisher must submit explanation of change with this statement)

PS Form 3526, July 2014 [Page 1 of 4 (see instructions page 4)] PSN: 7530-01-000-9931 PRIVACY NOTICE: See our privacy policy on www.usps.com.

13. Publication Title	14. Issue Date for Circulation Data Below
IMMUNOLOGY AND ALLERGY CLINICS OF NORTH AMERICA	MAY 2020

15. Extent and Nature of Circulation		Average No. Copies Each Issue During Preceding 12 Months	No. Copies of Single Issue Published Nearest to Filing Date
a. Total Number of Copies (Net press run)		143	128
b. Paid Circulation (By Mail and Outside the Mail)	(1) Mailed Outside-County Paid Subscriptions Stated on PS Form 3541 (Include paid distribution above nominal rate, advertiser's proof copies, and exchange copies)	87	78
	(2) Mailed In-County Paid Subscriptions Stated on PS Form 3541 (Include paid distribution above nominal rate, advertiser's proof copies, and exchange copies)	0	0
	(3) Paid Distribution Outside the Mails Including Sales Through Dealers and Carriers, Street Vendors, Counter Sales, and Other Paid Distribution Outside USPS®	26	21
	(4) Paid Distribution by Other Classes of Mail Through the USPS (e.g. First-Class Mail®)	0	0
c. Total Paid Distribution (Sum of 15b (1), (2), (3), and (4))	▶	113	99
d. Free or Nominal Rate Distribution (By Mail and Outside the Mail)	(1) Free or Nominal Rate Outside-County Copies included on PS Form 3541	16	14
	(2) Free or Nominal Rate In-County Copies Included on PS Form 3541	0	0
	(3) Free or Nominal Rate Copies Mailed at Other Classes Through the USPS (e.g. First-Class Mail)	0	0
	(4) Free or Nominal Rate Distribution Outside the Mail (Carriers or other means)	16	14
e. Total Free or Nominal Rate Distribution (Sum of 15d (1), (2), (3) and (4))	▶	16	14
f. Total Distribution (Sum of 15c and 15e)	▶	129	113
g. Copies not Distributed (See Instructions to Publishers #4 (page #3))	▶	14	15
h. Total (Sum of 15f and g)	▶	143	128
i. Percent Paid (15c divided by 15f times 100)	▶	87.59%	87.61%

* If you are claiming electronic copies, go to line 16 on page 3. If you are not claiming electronic copies, skip to line 17 on page 3.

16. Electronic Copy Circulation		Average No. Copies Each Issue During Preceding 12 Months	No. Copies of Single Issue Published Nearest to Filing Date
a. Paid Electronic Copies	▶		
b. Total Paid Print Copies (Line 15c) + Paid Electronic Copies (Line 16a)	▶		
c. Total Print Distribution (Line 15f) + Paid Electronic Copies (Line 16a)	▶		
d. Percent Paid (Both Print & Electronic Copies) (16b divided by 16c × 100)	▶		

☒ I certify that 50% of all my distributed copies (electronic and print) are paid above a nominal price.

17. Publication of Statement of Ownership

☒ If the publication is a general publication, publication of this statement is required. Will be printed in the NOVEMBER 2020 issue of this publication. ☐ Publication not required.

18. Signature and Title of Editor, Publisher, Business Manager, or Owner

Malathi Samayan   Date 9/18/2020

Malathi Samayan - Distribution Controller

I certify that all information furnished on this form is true and complete. I understand that anyone who furnishes false or misleading information on this form or who omits material or information requested on the form may be subject to criminal sanctions (including fines and imprisonment) and/or civil sanctions (including civil penalties).

PS Form 3526, July 2014 (Page 3 of 4) PRIVACY NOTICE: See our privacy policy on www.usps.com

Moving?

Make sure your subscription moves with you!

To notify us of your new address, find your **Clinics Account Number** (located on your mailing label above your name), and contact customer service at:

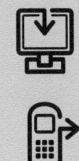

Email: journalscustomerservice-usa@elsevier.com

800-654-2452 (subscribers in the U.S. & Canada)
314-447-8871 (subscribers outside of the U.S. & Canada)

Fax number: 314-447-8029

Elsevier Health Sciences Division
Subscription Customer Service
3251 Riverport Lane
Maryland Heights, MO 63043

ELSEVIER